# DEJA REVIEW™

## Biochemistry  W9-BHM-734

# NOTICE

Medicine is an ever-changing science. As new research and clinical experience broaden our knowledge, changes in treatment and drug therapy are required. The authors and the publisher of this work have checked with sources believed to be reliable in their efforts to provide information that is complete and generally in accord with the standards accepted at the time of publication. However, in view of the possibility of human error or changes in medical sciences, neither the authors nor the publisher nor any other party who has been involved in the preparation or publication of this work warrants that the information contained herein is in every respect accurate or complete, and they disclaim all responsibility for any errors or omissions or for the results obtained from use of the information contained in this work. Readers are encouraged to confirm the information contained herein with other sources. For example and in particular, readers are advised to check the product information sheet included in the package of each drug they plan to administer to be certain that the information contained in this work is accurate and that changes have not been made in the recommended dose or in the contraindications for administration. This recommendation is of particular importance in connection with new or infrequently used drugs.

# DEJA REVIEW™
## Biochemistry

### Saad M. Manzoul

Case Western Reserve University
School of Medicine
Class of 2007

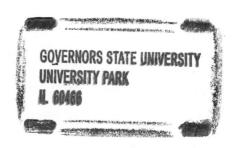
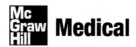 **Medical**

New York   Chicago   San Francisco   Lisbon   London   Madrid   Mexico City
Milan   New Delhi   San Juan   Seoul   Singapore   Sydney   Toronto

**The McGraw·Hill** Companies

# Deja Review™: Biochemistry

1 2 3 4 5 6 7 8 9 0  DOC/DOC  0 9 8 7 6

ISBN-10: 0-07-147463-3
ISBN-13: 978-0-07-147463-4

This book was set in Palatino by International Typesetting and Composition.
The editors were Marsha S. Loeb and Patrick Carr.
The production supervisor was Catherine Saggese.
Project management was provided by International Typesetting and Composition.
RR Donnelly was printer and binder.

This book is printed on acid-free paper.

International Edition ISBN-10: 0-07-110101-2; ISBN-13: 978-0-07-110101-1.

**Library of Congress Cataloging-in-Publication Data**

Manzoul, Saad M.
  Deja review : biochemistry / Saad M. Manzoul.
    p. ; cm. — (Deja review)
  ISBN 0-07-147463-3
    1. Biochemistry—Examinations, questions, etc.   I. Title.   II. Title: Biochemistry.
  III. Series.
    [DNLM:  1. Biochemistry—Examination Questions. QU 18.2 M296d 2006]
  QP518.3.M34 2006
  572.0076—dc22

                                                                    2006046676

*To Mahmoud A. Manzoul*
*—Saad M. Manzoul*

# Contents

# Faculty Reviewer

**Robert Haynie, MD, PhD**
Associate Dean for Student Affairs
Case Western Reserve University
School of Medicine
Cleveland, Ohio

# Student Reviewers

**Amanda Carlson**
Medical Student
University of Connecticut School of
Medicine
Class of 2007

**Brian Piltz**
Medical Student
University of Washington School of
Medicine
Class of 2006

# Contributing Authors

**Bruk Endale**
Medical Student
Case Western Reserve University
School of Medicine
Cleveland, Ohio

**Delwin S. Merchant**
Medical Student
Case Western Reserve University
School of Medicine
Cleveland, Ohio

**Anand Satyapriya**
Medical Student
Case Western Reserve University
School of Medicine
Cleveland, Ohio

# Preface

The *Deja Review: Biochemistry* book was designed for the student as a compact yet high-yield review of the major biochemical concepts necessary to master the subject in how it relates to medicine. As such, this book not only manages to cover the basic topics but also integrates pathophysiology and pharmacologic correlates with newly introduced material. We believe that along with the easy-to-understand figures, this book will serve as a great review and an important tool in assessing one's level of knowledge and achievement in biochemistry.

*Saad M. Manzoul*

# Acknowledgments

I would like to thank each of the contributors and Dr. Robert Haynie for their time and effort in organizing and reviewing the information contained in this book. For their knowledge and expertise throughout the entire process, I would like to thank Marsha Loeb and the entire McGraw-Hill staff.

I would like to thank the entire Manzoul family, Nagwa Taha, the Mohammed family, the Elhagmusa family, the Elbuluk family, and my friends for their unwavering support and encouragement.

# CHAPTER 1

# Proteins

## OVERVIEW

| | |
|---|---|
| How many amino acids make up mammalian proteins? | 20 |
| How do amino acids connect to make proteins? | Via peptide bonds (amino group bound to carboxyl group) |
| What is the basic structure of an amino acid? | See Fig. 1.1 |
| What are four classes of amino acid side chains? | Amino acids with nonpolar side chains |
| | Amino acids with uncharged polar side chains |
| | Amino acids with acidic side chains |
| | Amino acids with basic side chains |
| Name the amino acids with nonpolar side chains. | Glycine, alanine, valine, leucine, isoleucine, phenylalanine, tryptophan, methionine, proline |

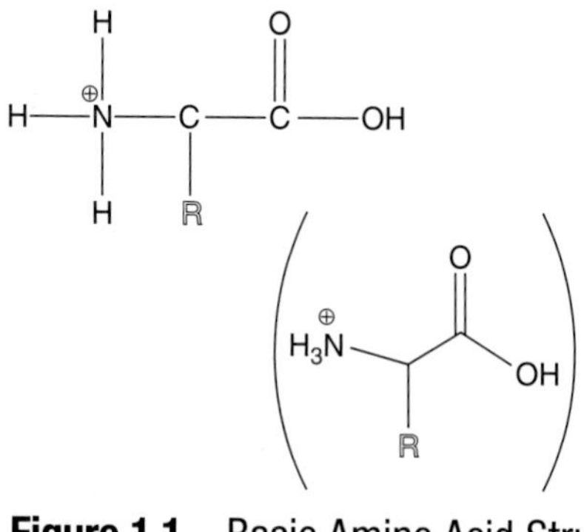

**Figure 1.1**   Basic Amino Acid Structure.

| | |
|---|---|
| **Name the amino acids with uncharged polar side chains.** | Serine, threonine, tyrosine, asparagine, cysteine, glutamine |
| **Name the amino acids with acidic side chains.** | Aspartic acid, glutamic acid |
| **Name the amino acids with basic side chains.** | Histidine, lysine, arginine |
| **What are the essential amino acids?** | PVT TIM HALL—phenylalanine, valine, tryptophan, threonine, isoleucine, methionine, histidine, alanine, leucine, lysine |
| **What is the Henderson-Hasselbalch equation?** | $pH = pKa + \log [A^-]/[HA]$ |

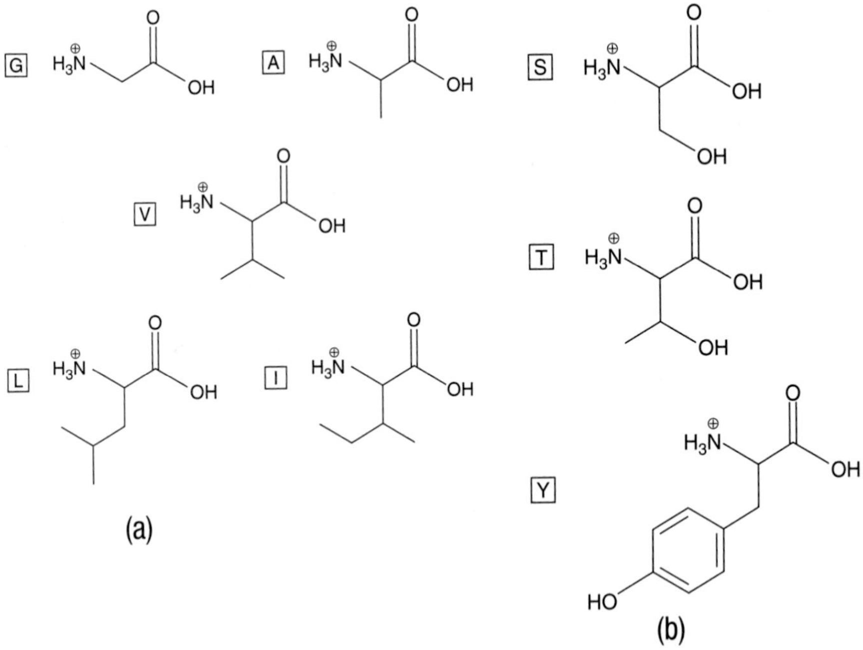

**Figure 1.2** Amino Acids. (a) Alipathic Side Chains (G—Glycine, A—Alanine, V—Valine, L—Leucine, I—Isoleucine); (b) Hydroxylic Group Side Chains (S—Serine, T—Threonine, Y—Tyrosine); (c) Sulfur-Containing Side Chains (C—Cysteine, M—Methionine); (d) Acidic Side Chains (D—Aspartic Acid, N—Asparagine, E—Glutamic Acid, Q—Glutamine); (e) Basic Side Chains (R—Arginine, K—Lysine, H—Histidine); (f) Aromatic Ring-Containing Side Chains (H—Histidine, F—Phenylalanine, Y—Tyrosine , W—Tryptophan); (g) (P—Proline).

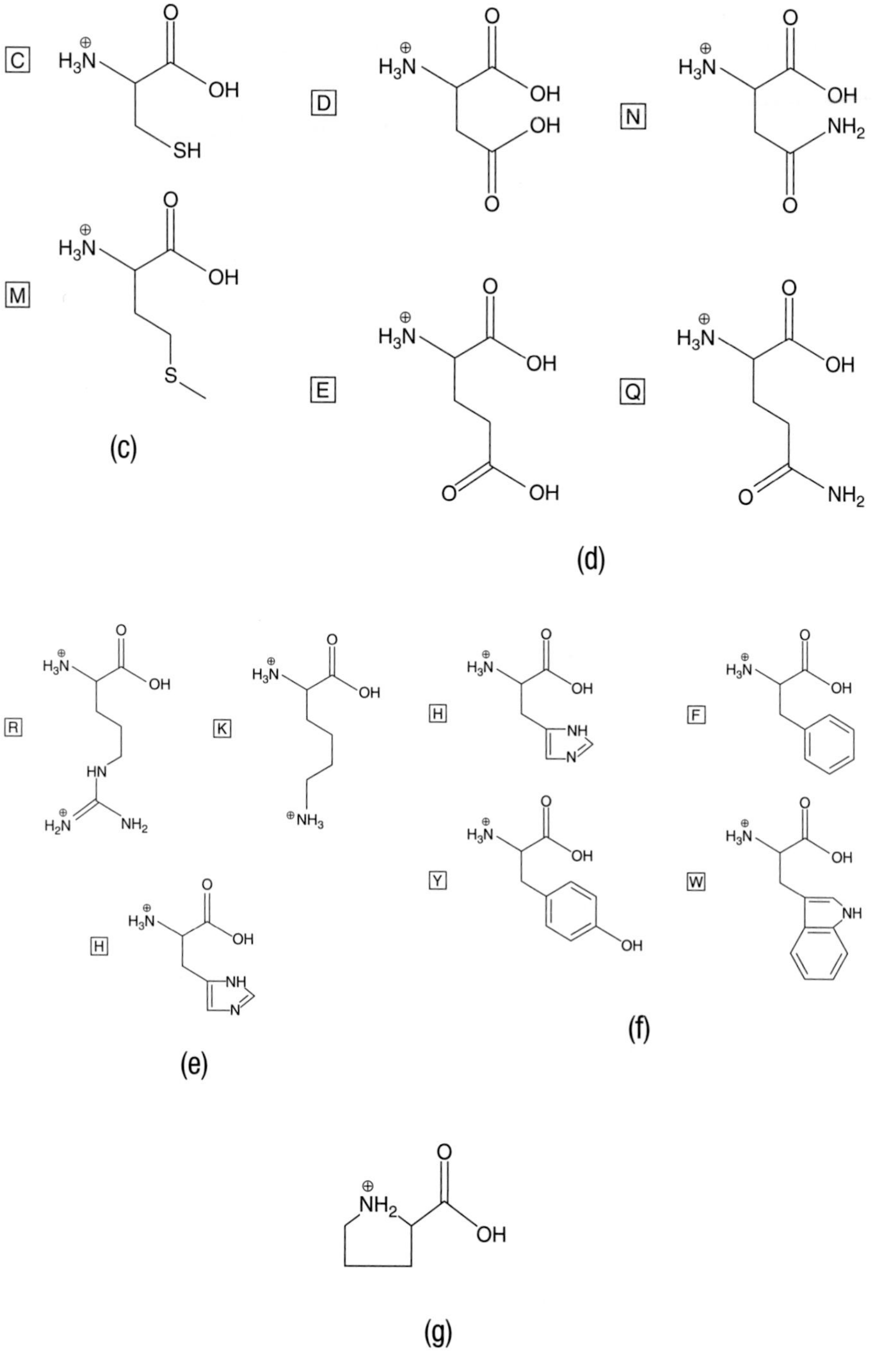

**Figure 1.2** (*Continued*)

| | |
|---|---|
| **How does this equation pertain to amino acids?** | At pH values greater than the p$K_a$, the carboxyl group of an amino acid loses its proton ($H^+$), $COO^-$; at pH values less then the p$K_a$, an amino group gains a proton ($H^+$) |
| **What is physiologic pH?** | 7.35–7.45 |
| **What is considered acidotic pH?** | Less than 7.35 |
| **What is considered alkalotic pH?** | Greater than 7.45 |
| **For amino acids with uncharged side chains, what is their overall charge?** | They are neutral at physiologic pH, due to the amino group being positive ($NH_3^+$), and the carboxyl group being negative ($COO^-$) |
| **At an acidic pH, what is the charge of an amino acid with an uncharged side chain?** | Positive due to the amino group gaining a proton ($NH_3^+$) |
| **At an alkalotic pH, what is the charge of an amino acid with an uncharged side chain?** | Negative due to the carboxyl group losing a proton ($COO^-$) |
| **What are the four levels of protein structure?** | Primary, secondary, tertiary, and quaternary |
| **What does primary structure mean?** | The sequence of amino acids in a protein |
| **What are the four characteristics of the peptide bond?** | Lack of rotation around the bond, planar, transconfiguration, uncharged but polar |
| **What is the secondary structure of a protein?** | The regular arrangements of amino acids |
| **What are the three most common types of secondary structure?** | $\alpha$-helix, $\beta$-sheet, $\beta$-bend |
| **Name two proteins in the body that are primarily $\alpha$-helical?** | Hemoglobin (80% $\alpha$-helical) and keratin (nearly entirely $\alpha$-helical) |
| **Name two properties of an $\alpha$-helix.** | Stabilized by hydrogen bonds between the peptide-bond carbonyl oxygens and amide hydrogens that are part of the polypeptide backbone; each turn of the $\alpha$-helix contains approximately 3.6 amino acids |
| **Which amino acids disrupt an $\alpha$-helix?** | Proline (inserts a kink in the chain), large numbers of charged amino acids (glutamate, aspartate, histidine, lysine arginine), amino acids with bulky side chains (tryptophan), or amino acids that branch at the $\beta$-carbon (valine, isoleucine) |

| | |
|---|---|
| **What is the difference between an α-helix and a β-sheet?** | An α-helix contains one peptide chain; a β-sheet contains two or more |
| **What are the forms a β-sheet can take on?** | They can either be parallel or antiparallel β-sheets |
| **Name a protein-like structure composed of primarily β-sheets.** | Amyloid |
| **In what disease processes is amyloid deposited within the body?** | Alzheimer's disease, multiple myeloma, Down syndrome, chronic hemodialysis |
| **What do β-bends do?** | They reverse the direction of a polypeptide chain to form a compact, globular shape |
| **Which amino acid is frequently found in β-bends?** | Glycine |
| **What does tertiary structure mean?** | The folding of domains, and the final arrangement of domains in the polypeptide |
| **What determines the tertiary structure of a protein?** | The primary structure (the sequence of amino acids) |
| **Name the four types of interactions that cooperate in stabilizing the tertiary structure of a protein.** | Disulfide bonds, hydrophobic interactions, hydrogen bonds, and ionic interactions |
| **What is the quaternary structure of a protein?** | The arrangement of the many subunits in a protein (if two subunits—dimeric, three—trimeric, and so on) |
| **What is protein denaturation?** | The unfolding and disorganization of a protein's structure |
| **What can cause the denaturation of a protein?** | Heat, organic solvents, mechanical mixing, strong acids or bases, detergents, and ions of heavy metals such as lead and mercury |

## HEMEPROTEINS

| | |
|---|---|
| **What are the two most abundant hemeproteins in humans?** | Hemoglobin and myoglobin |
| **What is the difference between hemoglobin and myoglobin?** | Hemoglobin is made up of four subunits, whereas myoglobin is made up of one subunit. Hemoglobin is found in red blood cells (RBCs) and myoglobin is found in muscle. Hemoglobin also has less affinity for oxygen than myoglobin. |

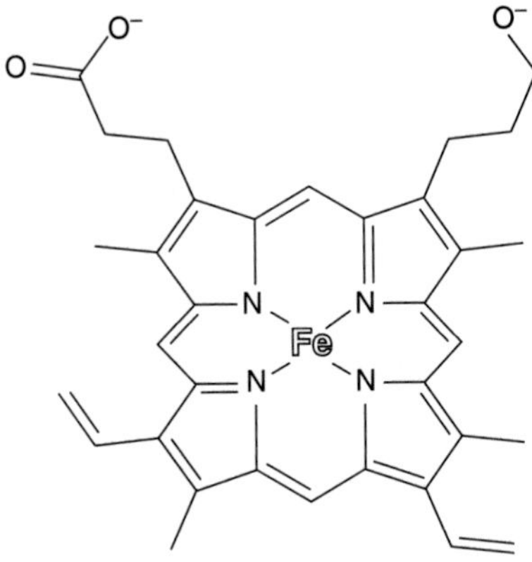

**Figure 1.3**   Heme.

| | |
|---|---|
| **What is heme?** | Heme is a complex of protoporphyrin IX and ferrous ion ($Fe^{2+}$) |
| **What enzyme catalyzes the rate-limiting step of heme synthesis?** | Aminolevulinate synthase, found in the liver and bone marrow |
| **How does lead cause microcytic, hypochromic anemia, and porphyria?** | Lead inhibits aminolevulinate synthase and ferrochelatase, thus preventing the incorporation of iron into heme. |

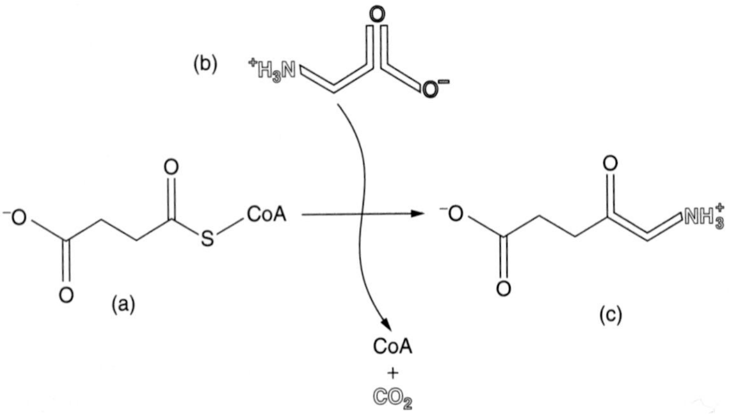

**Figure 1.4**   Heme Synthesis. (a) Succinyl CoA; (b) Glycine; (c) γ-Aminolevulinate.

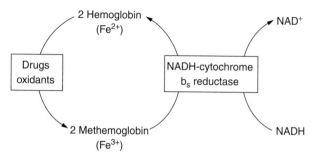

**Figure 1.5** Methemoglobin Synthesis.

| | |
|---|---|
| **What is methemoglobin?** | Hemoglobin with iron oxidized to $3^+$ (cannot bind $O_2$) |
| **What reduces methemoglobin ($Fe^{3+}$) to hemoglobin ($Fe^{2+}$)?** | Nicotinamide adenine dinucleotide (NADH)-methemoglobin reductase |
| **Why is methemoglobin used to prevent poisoning?** | Methemoglobin is used to prevent cyanide poisoning because it can avidly bind cyanide ion ($CN^-$), thus sequestering the cyanide ion and preventing it from inhibiting electron transport. |
| **Where is myoglobin often present in the body?** | The heart and skeletal muscle |
| **Where in the body is hemoglobin found?** | Exclusively in RBCs |
| **What is the function of hemoglobin?** | To transport oxygen from the lungs to the capillaries of body tissues |
| **What are the main types of hemoglobin?** | Hgb A = adult, Hgb F = fetal (many types), Hgb $A_2$, Hgb S = sickle cell (a mutant form), and Hgb C = crystal (a mutant form) |
| **What does Hgb A consist of?** | Two $\alpha$-chains and two $\beta$-chains ($\alpha_2, \beta_2$) |
| **What does Hgb F consist of?** | Two $\alpha$-chains like Hgb A, but two $\gamma$-chains instead of $\beta$-chains |
| **What are the two forms of hemoglobin?** | Taut (T, deoxygenated) and relaxed (R, oxygenated) |
| **What does cooperative binding mean in regard to hemoglobin?** | The binding of an oxygen molecule at one heme group increases the oxygen affinity of the remaining heme groups in the same hemoglobin molecule |

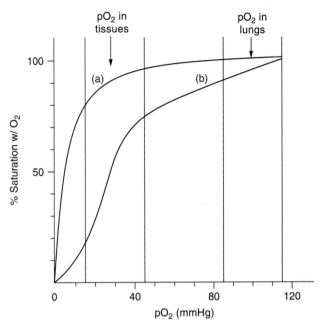

**Figure 1.6** Myoglobin and Hemoglobin Oxygen Dissociation Curves. (a) Myoglobin; (b) Hemoglobin.

| | |
|---|---|
| Does myoglobin bind oxygen in the same way that hemoglobin does? | No, because myoglobin has only one subunit |
| What is the significance of the sigmoidal shape of the $O_2$ dissociation curve? | This allows hemoglobin to carry and deliver oxygen efficiently from sites of high $O_2$ to sites of low $O_2$ |
| How is $CO_2$ carried in the body? | It is transported as bicarbonate ion, and carbamate bound to Hgb (minor form) |
| What variables shift the hemoglobin oxygen dissociation curve to the right? | Remember CADET Right:<br><br>Increased $CO_2$<br><br>Increased **A**cidity (decreased pH)<br><br>Increased 2,3-**D**PG (diphosphoglycerate)<br><br>Increased **E**xercise<br><br>Increased **T**emperature<br><br>Carbamate bound Hgb |
| What reaction does carbonic anhydrase catalyze? | $CO_2 + H_2O \rightarrow HCO_3^- + H^+$ (a reversible reaction) |

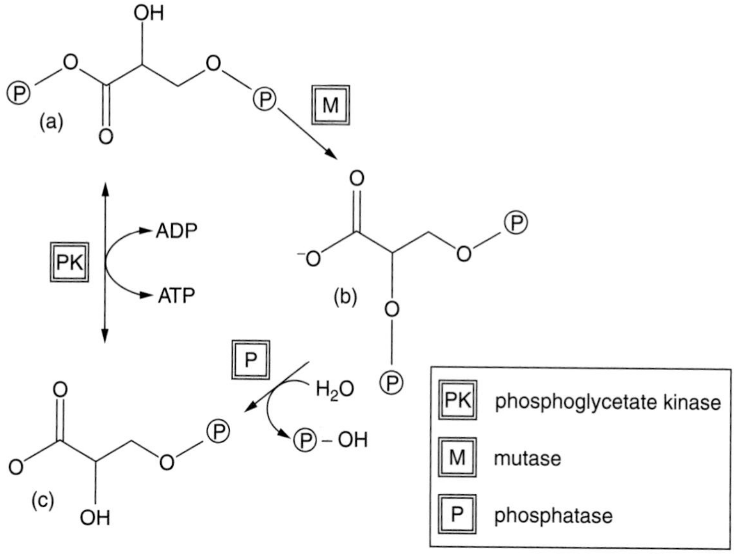

**Figure 1.7** 2,3-BPG Formation. (a) 1,3-Bisphosphoglycerate; (b) 2,3-Bisphosphoglycerate; (c) 3-Phosphoglycerate.

| | |
|---|---|
| **Describe the Bohr effect.** | The effect of $H^+$ concentration on the affinity of Hgb for $O_2$; as the $H^+$ concentration increases, the $O_2$ affinity decreases, causing a release of more oxygen to the tissue: |
| | Hgb $O_2$ (oxyhemoglobin) + $H^+ \rightarrow$ Hgb $H^+$ (deoxyhemoglobin) + $O_2$ |
| **How is the Bohr effect significant in $O_2$ transport?** | In the lungs, the pH is high, thus Hgb has high affinity for $O_2$ |
| | In the tissues, the pH is low, thus Hgb has low affinity for $O_2$ |
| **Where is 2,3-bisphosphoglycerate (BPG) created?** | In the glycolysis cycle from 1,3-BPG to 3-phosphoglycerate (PG) |
| **Does fetal Hgb or adult Hgb have a higher affinity for oxygen?** | Fetal Hgb |
| **What are the minor forms of hemoglobin?** | Hgb $A_2$ (appears about 12 weeks after birth, 2% of total Hgb); Hgb A1c (glycosylated Hgb) |
| **What disease process is Hgb A1c important in?** | Diabetes mellitus; glucose glycosylates Hgb and thus is a good marker of long-term glucose levels (RBCs have a life span of 120 days) |

**What are hemoglobinopathies ?**

A family of disorders caused by

Production of structurally abnormal Hgb

Synthesis of insufficient quantities of normal Hgb

Combination of both the above points

**What are the constituents of sickle cell Hgb?**

Two normal $\alpha$-globin chains and two mutant $\beta$-globin chains

**What is the mutation of the $\beta$-globin chain in sickle cell Hgb?**

Glutamate at position 6 replaced with valine

**What happens when RBCs sickle?**

They deform into a crescent shape, and frequently block the flow of blood in the small diameter capillaries (i.e., vasa recta of kidney, avascular necrosis of femoral head), thus causing anoxia (oxygen deprivation); this causes pain and eventual infarction

**What are some complications of sickle cell anemia (Hgb S homozygotes)?**

Aplastic crises (often due to parvovirus $B_{19}$ infection), autosplenectomy, *Salmonella* osteomyelitis, vaso-occlusive painful crises, nephropathy, and splenic sequestration crises

**Sickle cell anemia is most prevalent in what ethnic group in the United States?**

African Americans

**At what rate do African Americans carry the sickle cell trait?**

8% carry the Hgb S trait and 0.2% are Hgb S homozygotes

**What finding do you see on x-ray in individuals with sickle cell anemia?**

"Crew cut" on skull x-ray due to marrow expansion (also seen in thalassemias)

**What are some variables that increase the sickling of RBCs?**

Decreased oxygen, increased $CO_2$, decreased pH, increased 2,3-BPG, dehydration, deoxyhemoglobin S concentration

**Sickle cell heterozygotes have an advantage over nonsickle individuals in the presentation of what disease?**

Malaria (*Plasmodium falciparum*); sickle cell heterozygotes have a selective advantage in regions where malaria is a major cause of death

**Name some potential treatments for individuals with sickle cell anemia.**

Hydroxyurea (increases Hgb F), bone marrow transplantations, hydration, oxygen

**What mutation causes Hgb C?**

A single substitution in the sixth position of the $\beta$-globin chain (lysine for glutamate); these patients exhibit mild hemolytic anemia

**What mutation produces Hgb SC?**

One $\beta$-globin chain has the sickle cell mutation and the other has the C disease mutation; these patients have painful crises in their childhood but it is a milder disease than Hgb SS

**What is a common complication of Hgb SC disease?**

Deep vein thromboses (DVTs); Hgb SC patients are at a higher risk than the normal population and the sickle cell population to suffer from DVTs

**What are thalassemias?**

Hereditary hemolytic diseases in which an imbalance in the synthesis of globin chains occurs

**What is an $\alpha$-thalassemia?**

A condition in which the synthesis of the $\alpha$-globin chains (normally four) is decreased or absent

**How many different types of $\alpha$-thalassemias are there?**

Four, because there are normally four $\alpha$-genes

**What are the different types of $\alpha$-thalassemia?**

One of the four genes is defective = silent carrier

Two of the four genes are defective = $\alpha$-thalassemia trait

Three of the four genes are defective = Hgb H disease

All four genes are defective = Hgb Barts, Hydrops fetalis (fetal death occurs)

**What is a $\beta$-thalassemia?**

A condition in which the synthesis of the $\beta$-globin chains (normally two) is decreased or absent

**How many different types of $\beta$-thalassemia are there?**

Two, because there are normally two $\beta$ genes

**What are the different types of $\beta$-thalassemia ?**

One of the two genes is defective = $\beta$-thalassemia minor

Both of the genes are defective = $\beta$-thalassemia major

**In what geographical regions is $\alpha$-thalassemia most prevalent?**

Asia and Africa

| | |
|---|---|
| In which geographical region is β-thalassemia most prevalent? | Mediterranean |
| What type of hemoglobin is increased in β-thalassemia? | Hgb F |
| What is the treatment for β-thalassemia major? | Blood transfusion |
| What is a complication of this treatment? | Cardiac failure due to secondary hemochromatosis (increased iron from transfusions) |
| Characterize the anemia associated with thalassemia. | Microcytic, hypochromic anemias |
| What sign on x-ray is indicative of thalassemia? | "Crew cut" on skull x-ray due to marrow expansion (as in sickle cell anemia) |

## CONNECTIVE TISSUE PROTEINS

| | |
|---|---|
| Name the connective tissue proteins found throughout the body. | Collagen, elastin, and keratin |
| Where are these proteins located in the body? | Collagen and elastin are found in connective tissue, sclera, cornea, and blood vessel walls; keratin is found in skin and hair |
| What is the most abundant protein in the body? | Collagen |
| What is the structure of collagen? | Three polypeptides ($\alpha$-chains) wrapped around each other in a triple-helix formation |
| What is the sequence of amino acids in the triple-helix of collagen? | Glycine-XY (X and Y may be proline, hydroxyproline, or hydroxylysine) |
| What vitamin is required for the synthesis of collagen? | Vitamin C, required for hydroxylation of proline residues in collagen (technically vitamin C is not required for the synthesis of collagen, but posttranslational modification) |
| Deficiency of vitamin C is referred to as what disease? | Scurvy |

**Name some physical findings associated with this disease.**

Swollen gums, easy bruising, anemia, poor wound healing, weakness

**How is collagen synthesized?**

Specific prolyl and lysyl residues are hydroxylated (via prolyl hydroxylase—vitamin C, an antioxidant, regenerates the enzyme) in the endoplasmic reticulum, forming procollagen. Procollagen is exocytosed into the extracellular space. Procollagen is then cleaved to form tropocollagen, which then aggregates into collagen fibrils.

**What characteristic linking reinforces the structure of collagen?**

Covalent cross-linking of lysine-hydroxylysine residues between tropocollagen molecules

**Where is collagen type I located in the body?**

Bone, tendon, skin, dentin, fascia, cornea, late wound repair; 90% of collagen in the body is type I collagen (remember bONE)

**Where is collagen type II located in the body?**

Cartilage, vitreous body, nucleus pulposus (remember carTWOlage)

**Where is collagen type III located in the body?**

Reticulin fibers located in skin, blood vessels, uterus, fetal tissue, granulation tissue (remember reTHREEculin)

**Where is collagen type IV located in the body?**

Basement membrane or basal lamina (remember under the F(l)OUR)

**Where is collagen type X located in the body?**

Epiphyseal plate (remember cartilage calcifaTEN)

**Name three diseases with faulty collagen synthesis.**

Scurvy, Ehlers-Danlos, and osteogenesis imperfecta

**Name several signs of Ehlers-Danlos syndrome.**

Hyperextensible skin, tendency to bleed (easy bruising), hypermobile joints

**How many different types of Ehlers-Danlos syndromes are there?**

Ten types (including those with autosomal recessive, autosomal dominant, and X-linked recessive inheritance patterns)

**What significant vascular pathology is associated with Ehlers-Danlos syndrome?**

Berry aneurysms

**What is the most common mode of inheritance for osteogenesis imperfecta?**

Autosomal dominant

| | |
|---|---|
| **What are some signs and symptoms of osteogenesis imperfecta?** | Multiple fractures with minimal trauma, blue sclerae, hearing loss (abnormal middle ear bone formation), and dental problems (lack of dentition) |
| **Osteogenesis imperfecta may often be confused with what suspicion on the part of the physician?** | Child abuse |
| **Which type of osteogenesis imperfecta is fatal?** | Type II (fatal in utero or in the neonatal period) |
| **What serum protein inhibits elastin degradation?** | $\alpha$-1-Antitrypsin inhibits neutrophil elastase (a protease that acts in the extracellular space to degrade the elastin of alveolar walls and other structural proteins) |
| **Where is $\alpha$-1-antitrypsin produced?** | Primarily in the liver, by monocytes and macrophages |
| **What diseases are associated with $\alpha$-1-antitrypsin deficiency?** | Emphysema (barrel-chested individuals suffering from air trapping due to increased compliance but decreased elasticity) and liver damage (cirrhosis, cholestasis) |

## ENZYMES

| | |
|---|---|
| **What are enzymes?** | Protein catalysts that increase the rate of chemical reactions without being altered in the process |
| **Name six properties of an enzyme.** | Contains an active site |
| | Catalytically efficient |
| | Substrate-specific |
| | Utilizes cofactors |
| | Activity is potentially regulated |
| | Located in specific areas of the cell or extracellular space |
| **Does an enzyme change the chemical equilibrium of a reaction?** | No, it allows the reaction to take place at a faster rate |
| **Name the factors that can affect the rate of enzymatic catalysis of an enzyme.** | Substrate concentration, pH, and temperature |

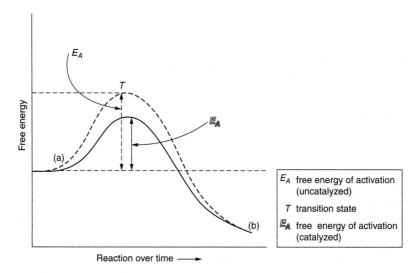

**Figure 1.8** Activation Energy and Enzyme Effect. (a) Initial State (Reactants); (b) Final State (Products).

**What is the effect of temperature on the reaction velocity?**

Increases with temperature until a peak velocity is reached and declines

**What is the effect of substrate concentration on reaction velocity?**

Increases with increasing substrate concentration until a maximal velocity is reached

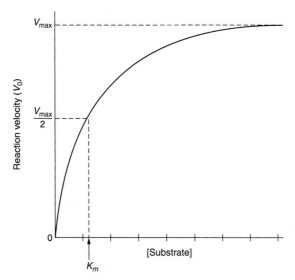

**Figure 1.9** Substrate Concentration vs. Reaction Velocity.

$$E + S \underset{k_{-1}}{\overset{k_1}{\rightleftharpoons}} ES \overset{k_2}{\longrightarrow} E + P$$

**Figure 1.10**   Enzymatic Action. (a) **E**—Enzyme; (b) **S**—Substrate; (c) **ES**—Enzyme-Substrate Complex; (d) $k_1$, $k_{-1}$, $k_2$—Rate Constants.

| | |
|---|---|
| **What is $V_{max}$?** | The maximum velocity at which an enzyme can catalyze a reaction (all conditions are optimal) |
| **What is the effect of pH on enzymatic activity?** | The catalytic process usually requires the enzyme ($E$) and substrate ($S$) to have certain chemical groups in an ionized or unionized state so they can react, i.e., some enzymes may require an amino group to be protonated ($NH_3^+$). Thus, at a high (basic) pH, the amino group is deprotonated and the enzyme-substrate ($ES$) complex cannot form; furthermore, extremes of pH can denature the enzyme. |
| **What is the Michaelis-Menten equation?** | $V_0 = V_{max}[S]/K_m + [S]$ |
| | $V_0$ = initial reaction velocity |
| | $V_{max}$ = maximal velocity |
| | $K_m$ = Michaelis constant |
| | $[S]$ = substrate concentration |
| **What does the Michaelis-Menten equation represent?** | The relationship between initial reaction velocity and substrate concentration |
| **What are the three assumptions of the Michaelis-Menten equation?** | $[S]$ is much greater than $[E]$ |
| | $[ES]$ does not change with time; that is, the rate of $ES$ formation is equal to the rate of $ES$ breakdown to either $E + S$ or $E + P$ |
| | Only the initial velocities are assumed |
| **What is $K_m$?** | $K_m$ is equal to the substrate concentration at which the reaction velocity is equal to $\frac{1}{2} V_{max}$ |
| **What does a small $K_m$ imply?** | High affinity of the enzyme for the substrate |

| | |
|---|---|
| **What does a large $K_m$ imply?** | Low affinity of the enzyme for the substrate, meaning a high concentration of substrate is needed to half-saturate the enzyme |
| **Does hexokinase have a large or small $K_m$?** | Low $K_m$, thus high affinity for glucose; it is saturated at normal blood glucose concentrations; hexokinase is found in most tissues |
| **Does glucokinase have a large or small $K_m$?** | High $K_m$, thus low affinity for glucose; it is saturated only at high blood glucose concentrations; glucokinase is present in only the liver and pancreas |
| **What is meant by the term *zero-order reaction*?** | The velocity of the reaction is constant and independent of substrate concentration |
| **What enzyme showcases zero-order reaction kinetics?** | Alcohol dehydrogenase in ethanol metabolism; you cannot speed up the reaction by adding more enzyme |
| **What is meant by the term *first-order reaction*?** | The reaction is directly proportional to the amount of substrate, therefore a linear relationship |
| **How does a competitive inhibitor inhibit an enzymatic reaction?** | By competing with the substrate for the active site on an enzyme |
| **Can the effect of a competitive inhibitor be overcome by increasing the amount of substrate?** | Yes |
| **What is the effect of a competitive inhibitor on the Michaelis-Menten equation?** | Increases the apparent $K_m$, but $V_{max}$ remains the same |
| **How does a noncompetitive inhibitor inhibit an enzymatic reaction?** | By binding to an allosteric site (not at the active site) on the enzyme |
| **Can the effect of a noncompetitive inhibitor be overcome by increasing the amount of substrate?** | No |
| **What is the effect of a noncompetitive inhibitor on the Michaelis-Menten equation?** | Decreases the $V_{max}$, but the $K_m$ remains the same |
| **How does a mixed inhibitor inhibit an enzymatic reaction?** | By binding to an allosteric site outside of the active site on an enzyme |
| **What is the effect of a mixed inhibitor on the Michaelis-Menten equation?** | Increases the $K_m$ and decreases the $V_{max}$ |

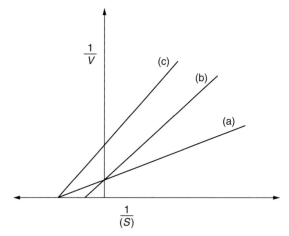

**Figure 1.11**   Lineweaver-Burke Plot. (a) Uninhibited;
(b) Competitive Inhibitor; (c) Noncompetitive Inhibitor.

| | |
|---|---|
| How does an uncompetitive inhibitor inhibit an enzymatic reaction? | By binding only to the $ES$ complex at an allosteric site |
| What is the effect of an uncompetitive inhibitor on the Michaelis-Menten equation? | Both the $V_{max}$ and the $K_m$ are changed |
| What is the only class of inhibitors that binds to the enzymatic active site? | Competitive inhibitors |
| What is the treatment for ethylene glycol poisoning? | Ethanol, because it is a competitive inhibitor of alcohol dehydrogenase (this decreases the production of toxic ethylene glycol metabolites); also fomepizole, hemodialysis, and gastric lavage |
| What can be a manifestation of ethylene glycol poisoning? | Kidney failure; ethylene glycol is oxidized via alcohol dehydrogenase to glycoaldehyde, oxalate, and lactate and later the oxalate crystallizes and deposits in the kidney |
| What is the treatment for methanol poisoning? | Ethanol, because it is a competitive inhibitor of alcohol dehydrogenase (this decreases the production of toxic methanol metabolites); also hemodialysis and gastric lavage |
| What can be a manifestation of methanol poisoning? | Blindness (optic atrophy); methanol is oxidized via alcohol dehydrogenase to formaldehyde and formic acid, to which the eyes are very sensitive |

| | |
|---|---|
| Name the methods the body uses to regulate enzyme activity. | Allosteric regulation, covalent modification, cofactor utilization, and induction/repression of enzyme synthesis; also proteolytic destruction of the enzyme |
| Describe the mechanism behind allosteric regulation. | An effector (i.e., a molecule) binds to the enzyme at an allosteric position and alters the activity of the enzyme |
| Allosteric regulation of enzymatic activity is associated with what type of substrate-velocity curve? | Sigmoidal, due to positive cooperativity (the binding of one substrate molecule facilitates the binding of other substrate molecules at other sites, similar to the hemoglobin dissociation curve) |
| What is the effect of a positive effector on the Michaelis-Menten equation? | Decreases the $K_m$, thus increasing the affinity of the enzyme for the substrate |
| What is the effect of a negative effector on the Michaelis-Menten equation? | Increases the $K_m$, thus decreasing the affinity of the enzyme for the substrate |
| What is meant by the term homotropic effector? | The substrate itself serves as an effector |
| What is meant by the term heterotropic effector? | The effector is a molecule other than the substrate itself |
| Describe the mechanism behind covalent modification. | Altering the activity of an enzyme via the covalent bonding of another molecule to the enzyme; most often accomplished by the addition/subtraction of phosphate groups, thus the enzyme could be more or less active in the phosphorylated form |
| Describe the effect of covalent modification on the activity of glycogen phosphorylase and glycogen synthase. | Addition of a phosphate group to glycogen phosphorylase increases its activity, whereas the addition of phosphate to glycogen synthase decreases its activity |
| Name several enzymes whose activity is mostly altered via the induction or repression of enzyme synthesis. | Cytochrome P450 enzymes (often the molecules these enzymes detoxify induce their synthesis), glycolytic enzymes (insulin induces their production); also 3-hydroxy-3-methylglutaryl coenzyme A (HMG-CoA) reductase |
| What is a cofactor? | A small molecule essential for the action of an enzyme |

**List several enzymes that utilize cofactors.**  Pyruvate dehydrogenase complex, $\alpha$-ketoglutarate dehydrogenase complex (both utilize vitamins $B_1$, $B_2$, $B_3$, $B_5$, and lipoic acid as cofactors), pancreatic lipase (utilizes colipase as a cofactor)

## AMINO ACID DISORDERS

**What symptoms are associated with phenylketonuria (PKU)?**  Affected infants are normal at birth but eventually develop increased plasma phenylalanine levels within the first few weeks of life. This leads to mental retardation and impairment of brain development, fair skin, eczema, and a characteristic musty body odor.

**What enzyme disturbances are associated with PKU?**  Decreased phenylalanine hydroxylase or decreased tetrahydrobiopterin cofactor, leading to decreased tyrosine production

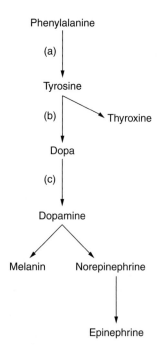

**Figure 1.12**   Phenylalanine Metabolism. (a) Phenylalanine Hydroxylase; (b) Tyrosine Hydroxylase; (c) Dopa Decarboxylase.

**What substances are found in increased amounts in the urine of those with PKU?**

Phenylketones (i.e., phenyllactate, phenylpyruvate, phenylacetate)

**When is PKU screened?**

At birth

**PKU is inherited in what pattern?**

Autosomal recessive

**What is the treatment for PKU?**

Decreased phenylalanine, increased tyrosine in the diet

**What is maternal PKU?**

This occurs when a mother's uncontrolled hyperphenylalaninemia leads to mental retardation and birth defects in the fetus as a result of phenylalanine crossing the placenta and interfering with organogenesis during weeks 3–8 of gestation. It may occur even if the fetus is not deficient in phenylalanine hydroxylase or tetrahydrobiopterin cofactor.

**Describe the pathophysiology behind maple syrup urine disease.**

Degradation of branched amino acids (i.e., isoleucine, valine, leucine) is blocked, thus causing increased $\alpha$-ketoacids in the blood

**What is the deficient enzyme in maple syrup urine disease?**

$\alpha$-Ketoacid dehydrogenase (cofactor thiamine)

**What are the symptoms of maple syrup urine disease?**

Mental retardation, edema, white matter demyelination, hyperglycemia, and death

**What pathophysiological processes can result in albinism?**

Deficiency of tyrosinase

Defective tyrosine transporters (which decreases the amount of melanin)

Lack of migration of neural crest cells

**What is the role of tyrosinase?**

Aids in the conversion of tyrosine to melanin

**What is the role of melanin?**

Gives pigment to the hair, skin, and iris

**What important pathology is associated with a decrease in melanin?**

Increased susceptibility to sunburns with an increased risk of developing squamous cell carcinoma

**Describe the pathophysiology behind homocystinuria.**

Defective cystathionine synthase and/or methionine synthase resulting in excess homocystine in the urine

**Describe the two forms of homocystinuria.**

Deficiency of either of the aforementioned enzymes

Decreased affinity of either enzyme for pyridoxal phosphate (vitamin $B_6$)

| | |
|---|---|
| **What is the treatment for the first form?** | Increased cysteine (because cysteine becomes an essential amino acid) and decreased methionine (because there is an accumulation of methionine and its metabolites in the blood) in the diet |
| **What is the treatment for the second form?** | Increased vitamin $B_6$ in the diet |
| **What are the symptoms of homocystinuria?** | Marfan-like body habitus (i.e., tall stature with long extremities, hyperextensive joints, long and tapering fingers and toes, lens dislocations), mental retardation, osteoporosis, thrombotic episodes (as a result of homocysteine damaging the vascular endothelium) |
| **What physiological defect is found in cystinuria?** | Defective renal tubular amino acid transporter for cystine, ornithine, lysine, and arginine (i.e., COLA) |
| **What major symptom is associated with cystinuria?** | Cystine kidney stones (radiolucent stones seen via imaging, yellow-brown hexagonal crystals seen macroscopically) |
| **What is the treatment for cystinuria?** | Acetazolamide (to alkalinize the urine and allow further excretion of cystine) |
| **What is the incidence of cystinuria?** | About 1:7000, important because it is the most common genetic error of amino acid transport |
| **What is the deficient enzyme in alkaptonuria?** | Homogentisic acid oxidase |

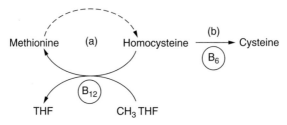

**Figure 1.13** Homocysteine Metabolism. (a) Methionine Synthase; (b) Cystathionine Synthase.

| | |
|---|---|
| The above enzyme is utilized in the degradation of what amino acid? | Tyrosine |
| What are the symptoms of alkaptonuria? | Generally no symptoms other than dark urine and connective tissue (onchronosis), although rarely some have severe arthralgias |
| What causes the urine and connective tissue to be dark? | Homogentisic acid accumulates, forming polymers (alkapton bodies), which causes the urine and connective tissue to darken |
| What is the prevalence of alkaptonuria? | 1:250,000 |
| What is the deficient enzyme in cystathioninuria? | Cystathionase |
| What reaction does cystathionase catalyze? | Formation of cysteine and α-ketobutyrate from cystathionine |
| What are the symptoms of cystathioninuria? | No clinical symptoms |
| What is the deficient enzyme in histidinemia? | Histidase |
| What reaction does this enzyme catalyze? | Histidine to urocanate |
| What are the symptoms of histidinemia? | Often asymptomatic, but mental retardation may be present |
| Describe the pathophysiology behind histidinemia. | Symptoms occur due to increased levels of histidine in the blood and urine |
| What inheritance pattern is seen in histidinemia? | Autosomal recessive |
| What is the prevalence of histidinemia? | 1:10,000 |

# CHAPTER 2

# Metabolism

## OVERVIEW

| | |
|---|---|
| What are the three major classes of carbohydrates? | Monosaccharides, disaccharides, and polysaccharides |
| What is the simplest of these carbohydrates? | Monosaccharides |
| What is the major fuel source of the brain? | Glucose |
| What are the major metabolic pathway(s) of the brain? | Glycolysis and amino acid metabolism |
| What cells do not contain mitochondria and thus rely only on glycolysis for energy production? | Erythrocytes |
| What type of tissue stores, synthesizes, and mobilizes triglycerides? | Adipose tissue |
| Which metabolic pathway does fast-twitch muscle use for fuel? | Glycolysis |
| Which metabolic pathway does slow-twitch muscle use for fuel? | Tricarboxylic acid (TCA) cycle and $\beta$-oxidation (i.e., aerobic pathways) |

## GLYCOLYSIS

| | |
|---|---|
| Name the family of glucose carrier proteins that transport glucose into the cell. | The GLUT proteins |
| What glucose transporter is used by the liver? | GLUT2 |
| What glucose transporter is used by muscle? | GLUT4 |
| Which one of the above transporters is sensitive to insulin? | GLUT4 |

| | |
|---|---|
| What is the mechanism of action of insulin on this transporter? | Facilitates movement of the receptor to cell membrane |
| What glucose transporter is located on the brush-border membrane of both intestinal and kidney cells? | S-GLUT |
| The above enzyme is coupled to the transport of what ion to provide energy for glucose transport? | $Na^+$ |
| In most tissues, glucose is trapped in the cell by phosphorylation by what enzyme? | Hexokinase |
| What inhibits the above enzyme? | Feedback inhibition by its product glucose-6-phosphate |
| In the liver, glucose is phosphorylated by what enzyme? | Glucokinase |
| What is the major distinction between hexokinase and glucokinase? | Glucokinase differs from hexokinase in that it requires a much larger glucose concentration ($K_m$) to achieve half saturation. |
| Does glucokinase or hexokinase prevent hyperglycemia following a carbohydrate-rich meal? | Glucokinase functions to prevent hyperglycemia following a carbohydrate-rich meal. |
| Which two organs express glucokinase? | Liver and pancreas |
| Describe the kinetics of glucokinase. | It has a high $K_m$ and high $V_{max}$ and is not subject to feedback inhibition by glucose-6-phosphate. |
| Describe the kinetics of hexokinase. | It has a low $K_m$ and low $V_{max}$ and is subject to feedback inhibition by glucose-6-phosphate. |
| What is the effect of insulin on this glucokinase? | Insulin induces synthesis of the glucokinase |
| Name two functions of glycolysis. | Degrading glucose to generate adenosine triphosphate (ATP) Providing building blocks for synthetic reactions (such as the formation of long-chain fatty acids) |
| How much ATP is consumed per mole of glucose that undergoes glycolysis? | 2 moles are consumed |
| How much ATP is generated per mole of glucose that undergoes glycolysis? | 4 moles |
| What is the net generation of ATP per mole of glucose that undergoes glycolysis? | 2 moles |

| | |
|---|---|
| **What is the major regulatory enzyme in glycolysis?** | Phosphofructokinase-I (PFK-I) |
| **Name the three enzymes of glycolysis that catalyze virtually irreversible reactions?** | Hexokinase, PFK-I, and pyruvate kinase |
| **What reaction does PFK-I catalyze?** | Fructose-6-phosphate $\rightarrow$ fructose-1, 6-bisphosphate (coupled to the hydrolysis of ATP) |
| **Name a positive allosteric regulator of this enzyme.** | Adenosine monophosphate (AMP), fructose-2,6-bisphosphate |
| **Name an allosteric inhibitor of this enzyme.** | ATP, citrate |
| **A deficiency in PFK-I results in what disease?** | Tarui disease |
| **What reaction does PFK-II catalyze?** | Fructose-6-phosphate $\rightarrow$ fructose-2, 6-bisphosphate |
| **In what organ is PFK-II not regulated by phosphorylation?** | Muscle |
| **Is activity of PFK-II a sign of the fed or fasting state?** | Fed state |
| **Which two glycolytic intermediates liberate enough energy for driving ATP synthesis?** | 1,3-Bisphosphoglycerate and phosphoenolpyruvate (PEP) |
| **What are the two ATP-producing enzymes of glycolysis?** | 3-Phosphoglycerate kinase and pyruvate kinase (think kinase) |
| **Pyruvate kinase catalyzes what reaction?** | PEP $\rightarrow$ pyruvate |
| **What covalent modification inhibits pyruvate kinase?** | Phosphorylation |
| **What enzyme carries out the above allosteric inhibition?** | Protein kinase A |
| **Name the allosteric inhibitors of pyruvate kinase.** | ATP, acetyl coenzyme (CoA); alanine in liver only |
| **Name the allosteric activator of pyruvate kinase?** | Fructose-1,6-bisphosphate |
| **What are the signs of pyruvate kinase deficiency?** | Anemia, reticulocytosis with macrovalocytosis, increased 2, 3-diphosphoglycerate (DPG) (remember red blood cells [RBCs] metabolize glucose anaerobically and thus depend solely on glycolysis) |
| **This disorder is inherited in what pattern?** | Autosomal recessive |

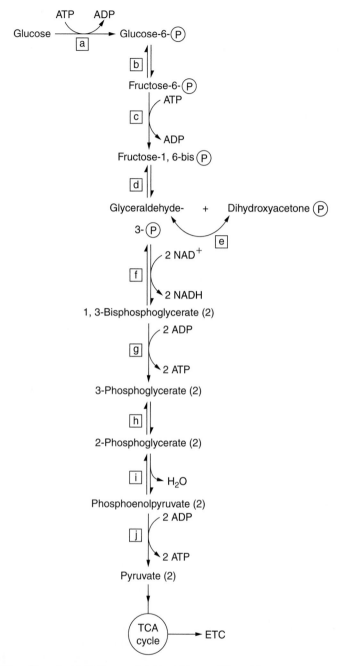

**Figure 2.1** Glycolysis Pathway. (a) Hexokinase/Glucokinase.
(b) Phosphoglucose mutase. (c) Phosphofructokinase I. (d) Aldolase.
(e) Triose phosphate isomerase. (f) Glyceraldehyde-3-phosphate dehydrogenase.
(g) Phosphoglycerate kinase. (h) Phosphoglycerate mutase. (i) Enolase.
(j) Pyruvate kinase.

| | |
|---|---|
| What is the most effective treatment for this disorder? | Exchange transfusions |
| Which enzyme produces nicotinamide adenine dinucleotide (NADH) in glycolysis? | Glyceraldehyde-3-phosphate dehydrogenase |
| How much NADH is produced per mole of glucose oxidized to pyruvate? | 2 moles |
| Since erythrocytes do not contain mitochondria, what is the NADH produced in glycolysis used for? | To reduce pyruvate to lactate |
| How is the reducing power of NADH transferred to the mitochondria? | Via the glycerol-3-phosphate shuttle or malate aspartate shuttle |
| What are the possible fates of pyruvate produced in the cell? | It can be converted to lactate, alanine, acetyl CoA, oxaloacetate, or glucose |
| How many moles of ATP are required to generate glucose from pyruvate? | 6 moles |
| Under anaerobic conditions, pyruvate is converted to what molecule? | Lactate |
| What enzyme catalyzes the aforementioned reaction? | Lactate dehydrogenase |
| What are the three enzymes of the pyruvate dehydrogenase (PDH) complex? | Pyruvate decarboxylase, dihydrolipoyl transacetylase, dihydrolipoyl dehydrogenase |
| What reaction does the PDH complex catalyze? | Pyruvate + $NAD^+$ + CoA $\rightarrow$ acetyl CoA + $CO_2$ + NADH |
| What coenzymes are required by this enzyme? | Thiamine pyrophosphate (vitamin $B_1$), coenzyme A (vitamin $B_5$), $NAD^+$ (vitamin $B_3$), flavin adenine dinucleotide (FAD) (vitamin $B_2$), and lipoic acid |
| The PDH complex is similar to what other enzyme? | $\alpha$-Ketoglutarate dehydrogenase complex |
| Is the PDH complex active in the phosphorylated or nonphosphorylated state? | Nonphosphorylated state |
| What enzyme phosphorylates the PDH complex? | PDH kinase |
| What molecules activate PDH kinase (thus inhibiting the PDH complex)? | Acetyl CoA, NADH |

| | |
|---|---|
| What molecules inhibit PDH kinase (thus activating the pyruvate dehydrogenase complex)? | Pyruvate, decreased levels of adenosine diphosphate (ADP) |
| What enzyme dephosphorylates the PDH complex? | PDH phosphorylase (PDH phosphatase) |
| What molecule activates PDH phosphatase (thus activating the PDH complex)? | $Ca^{2+}$ |
| What are the major manifestations of PDH deficiency? | Lactic acidosis, neurological manifestations |
| What is the treatment for PDH deficiency? | Increased intake of ketogenic nutrients |

## TRICARBOXYLIC ACID CYCLE

| | |
|---|---|
| For each acetyl CoA pushed through the TCA cycle, how much of the following molecules are produced: | |
| NADH? | Three |
| $FADH_2$? | One |
| $CO_2$? | Two |
| Guanosine triphosphate (GTP)? | One |
| How much ATP is produced per acetyl CoA pushed in the TCA cycle? | 12 ATP (2 × everything per glucose) |
| What reaction does citrate synthase catalyze? | Oxaloacetate + acetyl CoA → citrate |
| The presence of what molecule inhibits citrate synthase? | ATP |
| What reaction does isocitrate dehydrogenase catalyze? | Isocitrate + $NAD^+$ → $\alpha$-ketoglutarate + $CO_2$ + NADH |
| What molecules inhibit isocitrate dehydrogenase? | ATP, NADH |
| The presence of what molecule activates isocitrate dehydrogenase? | ADP |
| What enzyme catalyzes the formation of succinyl CoA from $\alpha$-ketoglutarate? | $\alpha$-Ketoglutarate dehydrogenase |
| This enzyme requires what cofactors in order to function? | Vitamins $B_1$, $B_2$, $B_3$, and $B_5$ and lipoic acid |
| The formation of succinyl CoA also releases what molecules? | NADH, $CO_2$ |

| | |
|---|---|
| **What molecules inhibit the aforementioned enzyme?** | Succinyl CoA, NADH, ATP |
| **The formation of what molecule in the TCA cycle results in GTP liberation?** | Succinate (via succinyl-CoA thiokinase) |
| **The formation of what molecule in the TCA cycle results in FADH$_2$ liberation?** | Fumarate (via succinate dehydrogenase) |
| **What reaction does malate dehydrogenase catalyze?** | Malate + NAD$^+$ → oxaloacetate + NADH |
| **Is the reaction that malate dehydrogenase catalyzes reversible?** | Yes (important in gluconeogenesis) |

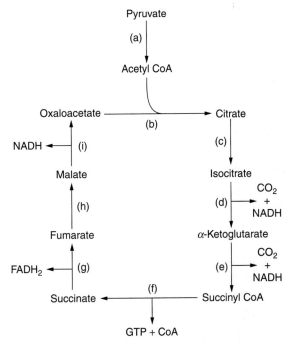

**Figure 2.2**  TCA Cycle. (a) Pyruvate Dehydrogenase; (b) Citrate Synthase; (c) Aconitase; (d) Isocitrate Dehydrogenase; (e) $\alpha$-Ketoglutarate Dehydrogenase; (f) Succinyl-CoA Synthetase; (g) Succinate Dehydrogenase; (h) Fumarase; (i) Malate Dehydrogenase.

# GLUCONEOGENESIS

| | |
|---|---|
| Where does the majority of gluconeogenesis occur? | Mainly in the liver, and to a lesser extent in the kidneys and intestinal epithelium |
| Name four substrates that can be used for gluconeogenesis. | Lactate, pyruvate, glycerol, and substances that can be converted to oxaloacetate (amino acid carbon skeletons) |
| Name four enzymes that circumvent the irreversible steps in glycolysis. | Pyruvate carboxylase, PEP carboxykinase, fructose-1, 6-bisphosphatase, glucose-6-phosphatase |
| Where in the cell can pyruvate carboxylase be found? | Mitochondria |
| What reaction does pyruvate carboxylase catalyze? | Pyruvate → oxaloacetate (which leaves the mitochondria) |
| Pyruvate carboxylase requires what coenzyme in order to function? | Biotin |
| What molecule in excess activates pyruvate carboxylase? | Acetyl CoA |
| Where in the cell can PEP carboxykinase be found? | Cytosol |
| What reaction does PEP carboxykinase catalyze? | Oxaloacetate → PEP |
| What triphosphate must be present in order for PEP carboxykinase to function? | GTP |
| What is the major manifestation of PEP carboxykinase deficiency? | Hypoglycemia afterfasting |
| Where in the cell can fructose-1, 6-bisphosphatase be found? | Cytosol |
| What reaction does fructose-1, 6-bisphosphatase catalyze? | Fructose-1,6-bisphosphate → fructose-6-phosphate |
| Where in the cell can glucose-6-phosphatase be found? | Cytosol |
| What reaction does glucose-6-phosphatase catalyze? | Glucose-6-phosphate → glucose |
| Glucose-6-phosphatase deficiency is also known as what disorder? | Von Gierke disease |

| | |
|---|---|
| In the aforementioned disorder, the liver becomes metabolically similar to what organ? | Muscle |
| What hormone is the main regulator of gluconeogenesis? | Glucagon |
| How does glucagon exert allosteric regulation on gluconeogenesis? | Glucagon decreases levels of fructose-2,6 bisphosphate, thereby activating fructose-1,6 bisphosphatase and inhibiting PFK. |
| How does glucagon regulate pyruvate kinase? | Glucagon increases levels of cyclic adenosine monophosphate (cAMP), which increases the activity of cAMP-dependent protein kinase. This causes pyruvate kinase to become inactive via covalent modification by the dependent protein kinase. |
| How does this mechanism alter the level of gluconeogenesis that occurs? | Decreasing the amount of active pyruvate kinase decreases the conversion of PEP to pyruvate, and diverts PEP toward glucose |
| How can a decrease in insulin alter gluconeogenesis? | Decreased insulin favors the mobilization of amino acids from muscle to the liver, which are used as carbon skeletons for gluconeogenesis |
| During starvation, which molecule acts as an activator of gluconeogenesis? | $\beta$-Oxidation of fatty acids during starvation increases the amount of acetyl CoA, exceeding the capacity of the liver to oxidize it to $CO_2$ |
| How does this molecule stimulate gluconeogenesis? | Excess acetyl CoA activates pyruvate carboxylase, increasing gluconeogenesis |
| Which by-product of exercising or ischemic muscle is used for gluconeogenesis? | Lactate |
| Which process describes the movement of gluconeogenic substrates between the muscle and the liver? | Cori cycle |

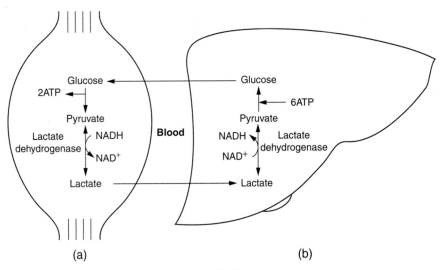

**Figure 2.3**   Cori Cycle. (a) Muscle; (b) Liver.

## OXIDATIVE PHOSPHORYLATION

**Where in the eukaryotic cell is oxidative phosphorylation (i.e., the electron transport chain, ETC) carried out?**

Across the mitochondrial inner membrane

**What reagents are involved in oxidative phosphorylation?**

Either NADH or $FADH_2$, which come from the TCA cycle

**What do the aforementioned reagents contribute to the ETC?**

Electrons

**What are the products of oxidative phosphorylation?**

$H_2O$; electrons are passed down the intermediates of the ETC and eventually reduce oxygen to produce $H_2O$

**What is the purpose of oxidative phosphorylation?**

To create a proton gradient by pushing $H^+$ into the mitochondrial intermembrane space, which then flows back into the mitochondrial matrix providing the energy to form ATP from ADP and $P_i$

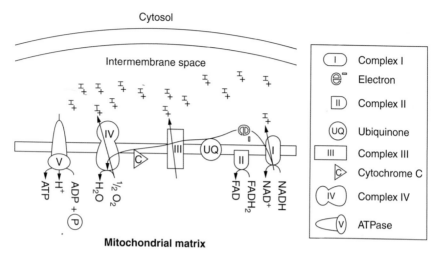

**Figure 2.4** The Electron Transport Chain.

**How is the ETC coupled with oxidative phosphorylation?**

The flow of ions into the mitochondrial matrix is considered to be oxidative phosphorylation, and the gradient is created by the ETC. Thus, these two processes are said to be coupled.

**How many molecules are involved in the ETC?**

Four complexes (Complexes I–IV) and two mobile electron carriers

**Name the two mobile electron carriers.**

Coenzyme Q (ubiquinone) and cytochrome c

**What is the name of Complex I?**

NADH dehydrogenase

**Electrons are transferred to Complex I of the ETC from what molecule?**

$NADH_2$

**What is the name of Complex II?**

Succinate dehydrogenase

**Where in the ETC does $FADH_2$ transfer its electrons?**

Complex II

**Describe the flow of electrons from NADH through the ETC complexes.**

NADH → Complex I → ubiquinone (coenzyme Q) → Complex III → cytochrome c → Complex IV → $O_2$

**Describe the flow of electrons from $FADH_2$ through the ETC complexes.**

$FADH_2$ → Complex II → ubiquinone (coenzyme Q) → Complex III → cytochrome c → Complex IV → $O_2$

**Which complex transfers its electrons to $O_2$?**

Complex IV

| | |
|---|---|
| Which molecule transfers electrons from Complex I to Complex II? | Ubiquinone |
| Which molecule transfers electrons from Complex III to Complex IV? | Cytochrome c |
| What is the only electron carrier that is not linked to a protein? | Coenzyme Q |
| As electrons pass through the complexes and the two mobile carriers, which push $H^+$ ions into the intermembrane space? | Complexes I, III, and IV (the others do not push protons into the intermembrane space) |
| How much ATP is produced ultimately from NADH traveling down the ETC? | ~3.5 ATP |
| How much ATP is produced ultimately from $FADH_2$ traveling down the ETC? | ~2 ATP |
| What enzyme synthesizes ATP in the inner mitochondrial membrane? | The $F_1F_0$ ATPase |
| The energy for synthesis of ATP is provided by what? | Movement of protons down their concentration gradient |
| Which domain contains the proton-conducting channel? | The $F_0$ domain |
| Which domain is the site of ATP synthesis? | The $F_1$ domain |
| Approximately how many $H^+$ ions does one turn of the $F_1F_0$ ATPase require? | 12–14 $H^+$ ions |
| What determines the rate of oxidative phosphorylation? | The availability of ADP |
| What is this type of regulation called? | Respiratory control, due to the fact that more ADP is created by increasing the metabolic rate (or *respiratory rate*), thus using up ATP and creating ADP |
| Name the inhibitors of Complex I. | Amobarbital (a barbiturate), rotenone (an insecticide), and piericidin A (an antibiotic) |
| Name an inhibitor of Complex II. | Antimycin A (an antibiotic) |
| Which oxygen analog inhibits the ETC? | Cyanide ($CN^-$) |
| Where does cyanide act in the ETC? | Complex IV |
| Name some other inhibitors of this complex in the ETC. | Hydrogen sulfide ($H_2S$) and carbon monoxide (CO) |
| What inhibits ATP synthesis by directly inhibiting the $F_1F_0$ ATPase? | Oligomycin |

| | |
|---|---|
| **Describe its mechanism of action.** | Oligomycin uncouples the ETC and oxidative phosphorylation by binding to the $F_1F_0$ ATPase; thus, oligomycin prevents the reentry of $H^+$ ions into the mitochondrial matrix and does not allow ATP to be formed. |
| **What agent inhibits oxidative phosphorylation by disrupting the proton gradient across the inner mitochondrial membrane?** | 2,4-Dinitrophenol (DNP) |
| **How does this molecule affect the proton gradient?** | Makes the inner mitochondrial membrane permeable to protons |
| **How does this molecule prevent the synthesis of ATP?** | Without a proton gradient, there is no energy for the $F_1F_0$ ATPase to utilize to combine ADP and $P_i$ |
| **With the use of ETC uncouplers, energy is dissipated in what form?** | Heat |
| **What molecule prevents ATP formation by inhibiting ATP/ADP translocation in the mitochondria?** | Atractyloside, thus preventing the formation of ATP |

## GLYCOGEN METABOLISM

| | |
|---|---|
| **What is the storage form of glucose in plants?** | Starch |
| **What breaks down starch in the body ?** | Starch is degraded by $\alpha$-amylase in saliva and pancreatic juice to maltose, triose, and $\alpha$-limit dextrans |
| **Where are disaccharides and monosaccharides degraded?** | Surface of epithelial cells in the small intestine |
| **By which process are monosaccharides absorbed?** | Carrier-mediated transport |
| **List the ways in which monosaccharides are utilized in the body.** | Oxidized to $CO_2$ and $H_2O$ for energy (via glycolysis/TCA/ETC) |
| | Stored as glycogen |
| | Converted to triglycerides (i.e., fat) |
| | Released into the general circulation as glucose |
| **In what form is glucose stored in the human body?** | Glycogen |

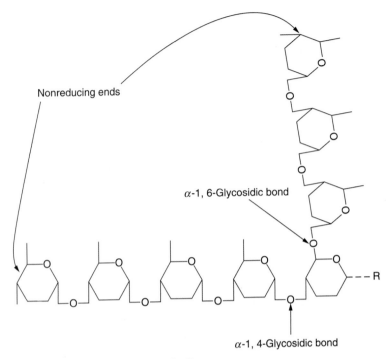

**Figure 2.5**  Glycogen Metabolism.

| | |
|---|---|
| **Where in the body does glycogen synthesis and breakdown occur?** | Liver and skeletal muscle |
| **What two types of linkages between glucose molecules may be found in glycogen?** | $\alpha$-1,4-Glycosidic bonds (between the glucose molecules placed in a straight line) |
| | $\alpha$-1,6-Glycosidic bonds (placed on the branch points) |
| **Where in the cell does glycogen synthesis take place?** | Cytosol |
| **What molecules provide the energy for the synthesis of glycogen?** | ATP and uridine triphosphate (UTP) |
| **What is the first step in the synthesis of glycogen from glucose?** | Glucose-6-phosphate $\rightarrow$ glucose-1-phosphate |
| **What enzyme catalyzes the aforementioned reaction?** | Phosphoglucomutase |
| **Uridine diphosphate (UDP)-glucose pyrophosphorylase catalyzes what reaction?** | Glucose-1-phosphate + UDP $\rightarrow$ UDP-glucose |

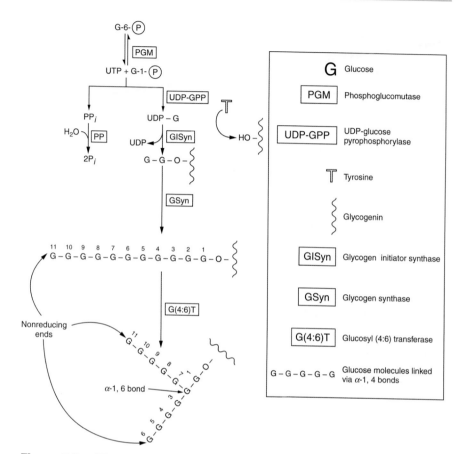

**Figure 2.6** Glycogen Synthesis.

What protein serves as the primer for glycogen synthesis?

Glycogenin

What reaction does glycogen initiator synthase catalyze?

UDP-glucose + glycogenin + glucose → UDP + linked glucose molecules

What enzyme is responsible for creating the α-1,4 linkage between glucose molecules?

Glycogen synthase

Can glycogen synthase initiate glycogen synthesis de novo?

No, it can only elongate an existing glycogen chain

Where on the newly synthesized glycogen chain are new glucose molecules added?

To the nonreducing end

| | |
|---|---|
| What would be the shape of a glycogen molecule if glycogen synthase was the only enzyme adding glucose molecules to the chain? | Linear |
| What enzyme is responsible for creating the $\alpha$-1,6 bonds between glucose molecules? | Glucosyl ($\alpha$-4:6) transferase |
| How does this branching enzyme work? | Transfers approximately 5–8 glucosyl residues from the nonreducing end of the glycogen chain to another residue within the chain and attaches the residues via an $\alpha$-1,6 linkage |
| What is the purpose of branching glycogen molecules? | To facilitate the breakdown of glycogen and aid in solubility |
| When is glycogen used as fuel? | During strenuous exercise in muscle; in the fasted state in liver |
| Is the process of glycogen breakdown the reverse of glycogen synthesis? | No |
| What enzyme is used to break down glycogen? | Glycogen phosphorylase |
| Where does glycogen phosphorylase cleave the glycogen molecule? | At the $\alpha$-1,4 glycosidic bond |
| How far away from the reducing end of the glycogen molecule can glycogen phosphorylase cleave? | Discontinues cleavage when there are four glucosyl residues remaining on a chain |
| What structure is the product of the above cleavage reaction? | Limit dextran |
| Can glycogen phosphorylase further degrade this product? | No |
| What enzyme removes glycogen branches? | Debranching enzyme complex |
| What are the two enzymes that constitute the debranching enzyme complex? | Oligo-($\alpha$-1,4 $\rightarrow$ $\alpha$-1,4) glucantransferase aka glucosyl (4:4) transferase; this enzyme removes the first three glucosyl residues left on a branch of glycogen |
| | Amylo-$\alpha$-(1,6)-glucosidase; this enzyme removes the last glucosyl residue on a branch of glycogen |
| Glycogenolysis liberates what glucose-based molecule? | Glucose-1-phosphate |
| What enzyme converts glucose-1-phosphate to glucose-6-phosphate? | Phosphoglucomutase (reversible action) |

| | |
|---|---|
| Which enzyme found on the endoplasmic reticulum of liver cells is responsible for liberating free glucose? | Glucose-6-phosphatase |
| What two mechanisms regulate glycogen synthase and glycogen phosphorylase? | Allosteric regulation and hormonal regulation |
| Which form of glycogen synthase, phosphorylated or nonphosphorylated, is the active form? | Nonphosphorylated |
| Which form of glycogen phosphorylase, phosphorylated or nonphosphorylated, is the active form? | Phosphorylated |
| Does glycogen synthesis occur in the fed or fasting state? | Fed state |
| Does glycogen breakdown occur in the fed or fasting state? | Fasting state |
| What hormone stimulates glycogen formation? | Insulin |
| What hormone stimulates glycogen breakdown? | Glucagon |
| In the well-fed state, what molecule allosterically activates glycogen synthase? | Glucose-6-phosphate |
| Name two molecules that allosterically inhibit glycogen phosphorylase. | Glucose-6-phosphate, ATP |
| In muscle, what effect does calcium have on glycogen phosphorylase? | Calcium binds calmodulin (a subunit of phosphorylase kinase) |
| | Phosphorylase kinase phosphorylates glycogen phosphorylase |
| | Phosphorylated glycogen phosphorylase is activated |
| | Glycogen is degraded to glucose (remember that when you need a boost in the muscle or more ATP, glycogen phosphorylase is activated) |
| In muscle, what is the effect of cAMP on glycogen synthase and glycogen phosphorylase? | cAMP inactivates glycogen synthase; cAMP activates glycogen phosphorylase |
| Describe the mechanism by which cAMP regulates glycogen synthesis. | Glucagon and epinephrine bind to their respective receptors |
| | Adenylate cyclase is activated and produces cAMP |
| | cAMP activates cAMP-dependent protein kinase |

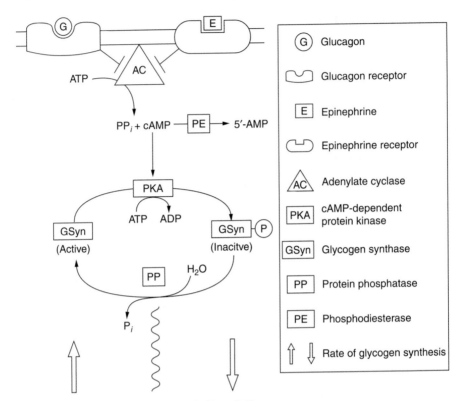

**Figure 2.7**  Glycogen Synthesis Regulation.

cAMP-dependent protein kinase phosphorylates glycogen synthase, thus deactivating the enzyme

cAMP-dependent protein kinase phosphorylates glycogen phosphorylase, thus activating the enzyme

**Name the common activators of glycogen phosphorylase.**

Glucagon, epinephrine; calcium and AMP in muscle

**Name the common inhibitors of glycogen phosphorylase.**

Insulin, glucose, ATP, glucose-6-phosphate

**Name the common activators of glycogen synthase.**

Glucose-6-phosphate, insulin

**Name the common inhibitors of glycogen synthase.**

Glucagon, epinephrine; calcium and AMP in muscle

**How many glycogen storage diseases are there?**

Twelve

| | |
|---|---|
| **What is glycogen storage disease type I called?** | Von Gierke disease |
| **What enzyme is deficient in Von Gierke disease?** | Glucose-6-phosphatase |
| **What are the symptoms of Von Gierke disease?** | Hypoglycemia, hepatomegaly, renomegaly, failure to thrive, stunted growth, hyperlipidemia, hyperuricemia, 50% mortality rate |
| **What is glycogen storage disease type II called?** | Pompe's disease |
| **What enzyme is deficient in Pompe's disease?** | Lysosomal $\alpha$-1,4 glucosidase (acid maltase) |
| **What are the symptoms of Pompe's disease?** | Mild hepatomegaly, cardiomegaly, widened QRS intervals on electrocardiogram (ECG), macroglossia, muscle hypotonia, cardiorespiratory failure within 2 years of life |
| **What is glycogen storage disease type III called?** | Cori disease |
| **What is the deficient enzyme in Cori disease?** | Debranching enzyme, $\alpha$-1, 6-glucosidase |
| **What are the symptoms of Cori disease?** | Hepatomegaly, slow growth, low blood sugar, sometimes seizures |
| **What is glycogen storage disease type IV called?** | Anderson's disease |
| **What is the deficient enzyme in glycogen storage disease type IV?** | Branching enzyme |
| **Describe the glycogen that would be found in the cells of an individual with glycogen storage disease type IV?** | Normal amount, but with very long outer branches |
| **What are the signs and symptoms of glycogen storage disease type IV?** | Liver cirrhosis with death before 2 years of age |
| **What is glycogen storage disease type V called?** | McArdle's disease |
| **What is the main organ affected in glycogen storage disease type V?** | Skeletal muscle |
| **What are the symptoms of McArdle's disease?** | Temporary weakness and cramping of skeletal muscles after exercise, normal mental development (increased glycogen in muscle), myoglobinuria with strenuous exercise |

| | |
|---|---|
| What is the deficient enzyme in McArdle's disease? | Skeletal muscle glycogen phosphorylase (remember the liver enzyme is normal) |
| What is glycogen storage disease type VI called? | Hers' disease |
| What is the deficient enzyme in glycogen storage disease type VI? | Phosphorylase (liver) |
| What are the signs and symptoms of glycogen storage disease type VI? | Mild hepatomegaly and hyperlipidemia |
| What is the deficient enzyme in glycogen storage disease type VII? | PFK |
| Describe the symptoms of glycogen storage disease type VII. | Painful muscle cramps with exercise |
| What is the deficient enzyme in glycogen storage disease type VIII? | Phosphorylase kinase (liver) |
| What are the symptoms of glycogen storage disease type VIII? | Mild hepatomegaly and hypoglycemia |
| All of the glycogen storage diseases show what inheritance pattern? | Autosomal recessive |

## DISACCHARIDE METABOLISM

| | |
|---|---|
| What enzymatic reaction does sucrase catalyze? | Sucrose → glucose + fructose |
| Where does the majority of fructose metabolism occur? | Liver |
| What is the first step in fructose metabolism? | Hexokinase converting fructose to fructose-6-phosphate in the muscle and kidney |
| Essential fructosuria results from a deficiency in what enzyme? | Fructokinase |
| What are the symptoms of fructosuria? | No symptoms, although fructose is seen in the blood and urine |
| What reaction does aldolase b (fructose-1-phosphate aldolase) catalyze? | Fructose-1-phosphate → dihydroxyacetone phosphate (DHAP) + glyceraldehydes |
| Hereditary fructose intolerance results from a deficiency in what enzyme? | Aldolase b |

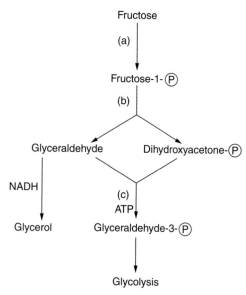

**Figure 2.8** Fructose Metabolism. (a) Fructokinase; (b) Aldolase b; (c) Triose Kinase.

| | |
|---|---|
| **Describe the pathophysiology behind fructose intolerance.** | The deficiency in aldolase b causes fructose-1-phosphate accumulation, thus sequestering phosphate molecules which results in decreased available phosphate. This decrease causes inhibition of glycogenolysis and gluconeogenesis. |
| **What are the symptoms of fructose intolerance?** | Jaundice, cirrhosis, hypoglycemia |
| **How is hereditary fructose intolerance treated?** | With a fructose (and sucrose)-restricted diet |
| **What are the possible fates of glyceraldehyde?** | Converted to glyceraldehyde-3 phosphate (an intermediate in glycolysis). Reduced to glycerol (to be used in fatty acid synthesis and gluconeogenesis) |
| **What reaction does lactase catalyze?** | Lactose → glucose + galactose |
| **What is the most common type of food intolerance?** | Lactase deficiency |
| **Where is the main site of lactase's action in the gastrointestinal (GI) tract?** | Small intestine |

**What are the symptoms of congenital lactose intolerance?**

Explosive, frothy stools, abdominal distention in infants exposed to milk or milk products; most experience diarrhea and malabsorption

**What is the primary dietary source of galactose?**

Milk

**Treatment of lactase deficiency with dietary lactose avoidance necessitates the supplementation of what electrolyte into the diet?**

Calcium

**What is the first step in galactose metabolism?**

Galactokinase converting galactose to galactose-1-phosphate

**What is the main purpose of the aforementioned step?**

To sequester galactose within the cell

**What reaction does galactose-1-phosphate uridyltransferase catalyze?**

It is involved in the conversion of galactose-1-phosphate and UDP-glucose to glucose-1-phosphate and UDP-galactose.

**UDP-galactose epimerase converts UDP-galactose to what?**

UDP-glucose (which cycles back for the above reaction)

**Is galactokinase deficiency or galactosemia associated with a more severe clinical course?**

Galactosemia

**List the signs and symptoms of galactosemia.**

Infants fail to thrive at birth and develop vomiting and diarrhea within a few days of milk ingestion. The most severely affected organs are the liver, brain, and eyes. Symptoms include hepatosplenomegaly, cirrhosis, cataracts, and mental retardation.

**What enzyme disturbance is associated with galactosemia?**

Absence of galactose-1-phosphate uridyltransferase

**What inheritance pattern is seen in galactosemia?**

Autosomal recessive

**What are the symptoms of galactokinase deficiency?**

Galactosemia in the blood and galactosuria in the urine; galactitol (a toxic metabolite of galactose metabolism) can accumulate if galactose is present in the diet; symptoms can include early congenital cataracts

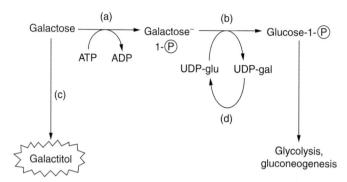

**Figure 2.9** Galactose Metabolism. (a) Galactokinase; (b) Uridyltransferase; (c) Aldose Reductase; (d) 4-Epimerase.

| | |
|---|---|
| What toxic metabolites are responsible for the clinical manifestations of the aforementioned disorders? | Galactitol and other galactose metabolites |
| Production of these toxic metabolites is the result of ectopic activity of what glycolytic enzyme? | Aldose reductase |
| What is the definitive treatment for these disorders? | Removal of galactose (and lactose) from the diet |

## HEXOSE MONOPHOSPHATE SHUNT

| | |
|---|---|
| What are the substrates for the pentose/hexose phosphate or hexose monophosphate (HMP) shunt? | Glucose-6-phosphate and nicotinamide adenine dinucleotide phosphate ($NADP^+$) |
| Where in the cell does the HMP shunt occur? | Cytoplasm |
| What organs in the body have extensive HMP shunt activity? | Lactating mammary glands, liver, adrenal cortex |
| What characteristic do these organs share? | Sites of fatty acid or steroid synthesis |
| What is the rate-limiting enzyme in the HMP shunt? | Glucose-6-phosphate dehydrogenase (G6PD) |
| Name an activator of the G6PD enzyme. | $NADP^+$ |
| Name an inducer of the G6PD enzyme. | Insulin |
| Name an inhibitor of the G6PD enzyme. | NADPH |
| What are the major products of the HMP shunt? | Ribose-5-phosphate and NADPH |

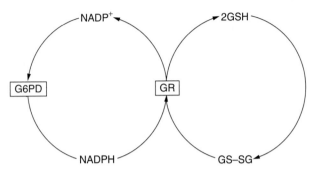

**Figure 2.10**   Glucose-6-Phosphate Dehydrogenase Pathway; G6PD
Glucose-6-Phosphate Dehydrogenase, GR Glutathione Reductase.

| | |
|---|---|
| **In what process is ribose-5-phosphate utilized?** | In nucleotide synthesis |
| **List three important processes which utilize NADPH.** | Anabolic processes (as a source of reducing equivalents) |
| | Respiratory burst |
| | Hepatic P450 function |
| **How do RBCs utilize NADPH?** | Via the glutathione reductase enzyme to reduce glutathione |
| **List four important processes which utilize glutathione.** | Reduction of protein sulfhydryl groups |
| | Reduction of peroxidases |
| | Maintenance of reduced hemoglobin (Hgb) |
| | "Catching" amino acids in the extracellular space (via $\gamma$-glutamyltranspeptidase) |
| **What steady-state cytoplasmic $NADP^+$/ $NADPH$ ratio favors redox reactions?** | 1/10 |
| **Why are RBCs particularly vulnerable to oxidative damage?** | RBCs have the capacity to carry large amounts of $O_2$, and are thus prone to oxidative damage because they have no ETC to reduce $O_2$. |
| **What type of oxidative damage can occur to the hemoglobin in RBCs?** | In the presence of reaction oxygen species (ROS), hemoglobin may precipitate to form Heinz bodies |
| **Heinz bodies are the histological hallmark of what disorder?** | G6PD deficiency |

What type of oxidative damage can occur to the plasma membranes of G6PD-deficient RBCs?

Peroxidation → membrane weakness → hemolytic anemia

What is the pathophysiology behind the symptoms of G6PD deficiency?

With deficient G6PD, NADPH is not regenerated, which leads to a decrease in NADPH and increase in $NADP^+$. Thus, less reduced glutathione is available to detoxify free radicals and peroxides. This results in the body's RBCs having a poorer defense against oxidizing agents, which leads to hemolytic anemia.

In what situations would oxidative damage in the presence of G6PD deficiency be accelerated?

Ingestion of foods containing oxidants (i.e., fava beans)

Treatment with certain drugs (i.e., sulfonamides, antituberculosis drugs)

Infections (i.e., pneumonia, infectious hepatitis)

In what ethnic group is G6PD deficiency most prevalent?

African Americans

Are males or females more likely to present with G6PD deficiency?

Males (X-linked recessive disorder)

How do polymorphonuclear leukocytes (PMNs) utilize NADPH?

NADPH is used by NADPH oxidase to produce ROS that destroy bacteria.

What is the most common cause of chronic granulomatous disease (CGD)?

NADPH oxidase deficiency in PMNs

What are the clinical manifestations of CGD?

Increased susceptibility to infection by catalase-positive organisms such as *Escherichia coli, Staphylococcus aureus,* and *Klebsiella;* increased risk of lymphoma

What test is used to confirm the diagnosis of CGD?

A negative nitroblue tetrazolium test

How do hepatocytes utilize NADPH?

In the biosynthesis of fatty acids, cholesterol, and nucleotides

## HEME METABOLISM

Name the two major sites of heme synthesis.

Bone marrow and liver

What enzyme catalyzes the rate-limiting step of heme synthesis?

Aminolevulinate (ALA) synthase

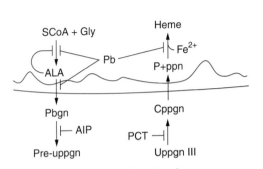

**Figure 2.11**  Heme Synthesis.

| | |
|---|---|
| What reaction does this enzyme catalyze? | Glycine + succinyl CoA → $\delta$-aminolevulinate |
| In what cellular compartment is this enzyme found? | Mitochondria |
| What molecule is the major inhibitor of this enzyme? | Heme (feedback inhibition) |
| Underproduction of heme results in what type of anemia? | Microcytic, hypochromic anemia |
| Define porphyria. | A group of disorders involving heme biosynthesis, characterized by the excessive excretion of porphyrins or their precursors |
| Describe the mechanism behind lead poisoning. | Lead inhibits ferrochelatase and ALA synthase |
| List six clinical features of lead poisoning. | Headache, nausea, abdominal pain, memory loss, neuropathy, lead lines in gums |
| What characteristic histological feature on a peripheral blood smear is found with lead poisoning? | Coarse basophilic stippling of erythrocytes |
| What two molecules accumulate in the urine in the setting of lead poisoning? | Coproporphyrin and ALA (urine may appear pink in color) |
| What is the enzymatic defect in acute intermittent porphyria (AIP)? | Deficiency in uroporphyrinogen I synthetase |
| What two molecules accumulate in the urine in AIP? | Porphobilinogen and $\delta$-ALA |
| Name three features of AIP. | Anxiety, abdominal pain, autosomal dominant inheritance |

What is the enzymatic defect in porphyria cutanea tarda (PCT)?

Deficiency of uroporphyrinogen decarboxylase

What molecules accumulate in the urine in PCT?

Uroporphyrin accumulates in urine, resulting in a tea color

What is the most common clinical feature of PCT?

Photosensitivity, resulting in inflammation and blistering of skin

How does bilirubin formation occur?

Heme is recovered from hemoglobin after hemolysis of RBCs in the spleen. This is subsequently converted to biliverdin, and then bilirubin.

How is unconjugated bilirubin transported in the blood?

Via albumin because bilirubin is not water soluble

What role do hepatocytes play in the metabolism of bilirubin?

Hepatocytes conjugate bilirubin with glucuronate via UDP-glucuronyl transferase, thus increasing its water solubility.

How does bilirubin enter the intestine?

Following conjugation, bilirubin is secreted into bile

How is bilirubin processed in the intestine?

Intestinal bacteria convert conjugated bilirubin into urobilinogen

How is bilirubin excreted in feces?

A portion of urobilinogen is converted into bile pigments (stercobilin) and excreted in feces

How is bilirubin excreted in urine?

A portion of urobilinogen is converted into urobilin (yellow) and is excreted in urine

What is jaundice?

A yellowish staining of the integument, sclerae, and deeper tissues and the excretions with bile pigments

Describe the types of hyperbilirubinemia, urine bilirubin, and urine urobilinogen levels in the following types of jaundice:

Hepatocellular

Conjugated (direct) or unconjugated (indirect) hyperbilirubinemia, increased urine bilirubin, normal or decreased urine urobilinogen

Obstructive

Conjugated hyperbilirubinemia, increased urine bilirubin, decreased urine urobilinogen

Hemolytic

Unconjugated hyperbilirubinemia, decreased/absent urine bilirubin, increased urine urobilinogen

| | |
|---|---|
| Name some hereditary hyperbilirubinemias. | Gilbert's syndrome, Crigler-Najjar syndrome, Dubin-Johnson syndrome, Rotor's syndrome, biliary atresia, and physiologic jaundice in the newborn |
| Which hereditary hyperbilirubinemias result from dysfunctional UDP-glucuronyl transferase? | Gilbert's syndrome, Crigler-Najjar syndrome |
| What type of hyperbilirubinemia is associated with these disorders? | Unconjugated hyperbilirubinemia |
| Which of the aforementioned disorders is typically asymptomatic? | Gilbert's syndrome (decreased UDP-glucuronyl transferase activity) |
| Which form of Crigler-Najjar syndrome is typically lethal early in life? | Type I |
| What are the signs and symptoms of this form of Crigler-Najjar syndrome? | Jaundice, kernicterus, increased unconjugated bilirubin |
| What is the treatment of this form of Crigler-Najjar syndrome? | Plasmapheresis, phototherapy |
| Which form of Crigler-Najjar syndrome responds to phenobarbital treatment? | Type II |
| Describe the pathophysiology behind Dubin-Johnson syndrome. | Defective liver excretion of conjugated bilirubin |
| What coproporphyrin I:coproporphyrin III ratio in the urine is characteristic of Dubin-Johnson syndrome? | 5:1 |
| On autopsy, will an individual who suffered from Dubin-Johnson or Rotor's syndrome have a blackened liver? | Dubin-Johnson syndrome results in blackened liver |
| What type of hyperbilirubinemia occurs with viral hepatitis or cirrhosis? | Conjugated and unconjugated hyperbilirubinemia, as well as increased aminotransferase (alanine aminotransferase/aspartate aminotransferase [AST/ALT]) levels |

## PURINE AND PYRIMIDINE METABOLISM

| | |
|---|---|
| Describe the structure of a nucleoside. | A nitrogenous base linked to a pentose monosaccharide |
| What differentiates a nucleoside from a nucleotide? | Addition of a phosphate group(s) |

| | |
|---|---|
| What bases make up the purine nucleotides? | Cytosine (C), uracil (U), and thymine (T) |
| What bases make up the pyrimidine nucleotides? | Adenosine (A) and guanine (G) |
| What compounds constitute the purine ring? | Amino acids (i.e., aspartic acid, glycine, glutamine), $CO_2$, and $N^{10}$-formyl-tetrahydrofolate |
| What enzyme catalyzes the rate-limiting step of the purine synthesis pathway? | Phosphoribosylpyrophosphate (PRPP) synthetase |
| What are the inhibitors of PRPP synthetase? | Inosine monophosphate (IMP), AMP, and guanosine monophosphate (GMP) |
| What is the rate-limiting step of the purine pathway? | Synthesis of 5-phosphoribosyl-1-pyrophosphate from ribose 5-phosphate |
| What is the committed step of the purine pathway? | Formation of 5′-phosphoribosylamine from 5-phosphoribosyl-1-pyrophosphate |
| The next several steps in the de novo purine synthesis pathway ultimately form what compound? | IMP |
| How many ATP molecules does this require? | Four |
| Upon synthesis of IMP, there is a fork in the pathway that leads to the formation of what two molecules? | AMP or GMP |
| What molecule is the energy source for AMP formation? | GTP |
| What molecule is the energy source for GMP formation? | ATP |
| Are AMP and GMP positive or negative regulators of their own synthesis? | Negative regulators |
| What enzymes are involved in the conversion of nucleoside monophosphates into nucleoside di- or triphosphates? | Adenylate kinase, guanylate kinase, nucleoside diphosphate kinase |
| What enzyme catalyzes the following reaction: AMP + ATP → ADP? | Adenylate kinase |
| What enzyme catalyzes the following reaction: GMP + ATP → GDP + ADP? | Guanylate kinase |
| Describe the reactions that nucleoside diphosphate kinase catalyze. | Interconversion of nucleoside diphosphates and triphosphates (i.e., GDP + ATP → GTP + ADP or CDP + ATP → CTP + ADP) |

| | |
|---|---|
| What drugs act to inhibit the conversion of $N^{10}$-formyl-tetrahydrofolate to tetrahydrofolate? | $p$-Aminobenzoic acid (PABA) antimetabolites (i.e., sulfonamides) and folic acid analogs (i.e., methotrexate) |
| What is the mechanism of action of PABA analogs? | Competitively inhibit dihydropteroate synthase, which leads to decreased bacterial synthesis of folic acid |
| Do these drugs affect human purine synthesis? | No, because humans cannot make folic acid |
| PABA analogs can be used to treat what bacterial infections? | Gram-positive, gram-negative, *Nocardia*, *Chlamydia* |
| What is the mechanism of action of folic acid analogs? | Competitively inhibit dihydrofolate reductase resulting in decreased trimethyl phosphate (dTMP), and thus decreased DNA and protein synthesis |
| What drug may be given to prevent toxicity from folic acid analog use? | Leucovorin (folinic acid) |
| What is the function of the purine salvage pathway? | To convert purines that result from cell turnover or from the diet; those that cannot be degraded are turned into nucleoside triphosphates |
| What are the three main enzymes involved in the purine salvage pathway? | Xanthine oxidase, HGPRT (hypoxanthine phospho-ribosyltransferase), and adenosine deaminase (ADA) |
| What disease is the result of ADA deficiency? | Severe combined immunodeficiency (i.e., SCID, an immunodeficiency in both B and T cells) |
| How does ADA deficiency cause this disease? | ADA deficiency causes an excess of ATP and dATP; this impacts negatively on ribonucleotide reductase and thus prevents DNA synthesis, which decreases B- and T-lymphocyte count |
| Does this disease most commonly present in childhood or adulthood? | Childhood |
| What types of infections are individuals with this disease likely to suffer from? | Recurrent viral, bacterial, fungal, and protozoal infections |
| What disease is the result of HGPRT deficiency? | Lesch-Nyhan syndrome |

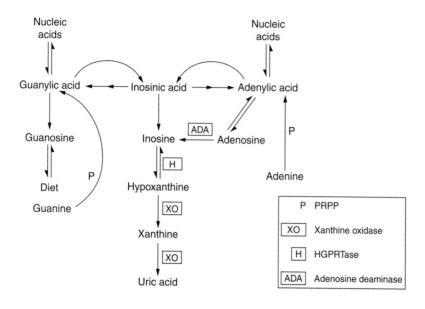

**Figure 2.12** Purine Salvage Pathway.

What are some findings associated with this disorder?

Mental retardation, aggression, self-mutilation, hyperuricemia, gout, and choreoathetosis

Serum levels of what substance are increased in Lesch-Nyhan syndrome?

Uric acid

What is the inheritance pattern of Lesch-Nyhan syndrome?

X-linked recessive

What is gout?

A disorder of purine metabolism characterized by a raised but variable blood uric acid level and severe recurrent acute arthritis of sudden onset resulting from deposition of sodium urate crystals in connective tissue and articular cartilage

Where is the characteristic location of an acute attack of gout?

Metatarsophalangeal joint of the great toe

Describe the sodium urate crystals.

Needle-shaped and negatively birefringent

List the possible causes of gout.

Lesch-Nyhan syndrome

PRPP excess

Decreased excretion of uric acid

G6PD deficiency

Administration of thiazide diuretics

**What is allopurinol's mechanism of action?** Xanthine oxidase inhibitor

**What substances have increased levels as a result of allopurinol's mechanism of action?** Hypoxanthine and xanthine

**Can these substances crystallize?** No

**What is the mechanism by which colchicine treats gout?** Depolymerizes microtubules and thus reduces inflammation by impairing leukocyte chemotaxis and degranulation

**What is the mechanism by which probenecid treats gout?** Probenecid inhibits the reabsorption of uric acid in the proximal tubule

**Which antigout drug delivers the most immediate relief following administration?** Colchicine

**What molecules provide the source of carbon and nitrogen atoms in the pyrimidine ring?** Glutamine, aspartic acid, and $CO_2$

**What is the committed step in pyrimidine synthesis?** Carbamoyl phosphate formation

**What catalyzes this reaction?** Carbamoyl phosphate synthetase II (CPS II)

**What cofactor is normally used in carboxylating reactions?** Biotin

**Does the aforementioned enzyme utilize this cofactor?** No

**In what other cycle is carbamoyl phosphate formed?** Urea cycle

**Name the key differences between CPS I and CPS II.** CPS I is involved in the urea cycle; CPS II is involved in pyrimidine synthesis

CPS I is in the mitochondria; CPS II is in the cytosol

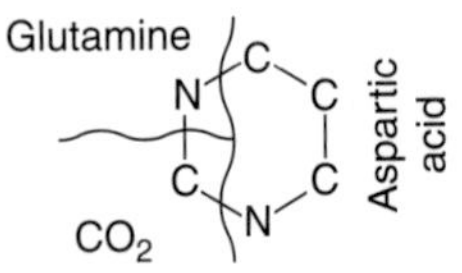

**Figure 2.13** Pyrimidine Constituents.

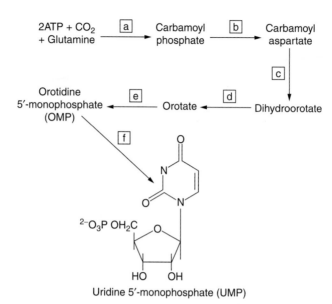

Uridine 5'-monophosphate (UMP)

**Figure. 2.14** Pyrimidine Synthesis. (a) Carbamoyl phosphate synthetase II; (b) Aspartate transcarbamoylase; (c) Dihydroorotase; (d) Dihydroorotate dehydrogenase; (e) Orotate phosphoribosyl-transferase; (f) OMP decarboxylase.

| | CPS I utilizes ammonia as its source of nitrogen; CPS II utilizes the $\gamma$-amide group of glutamate as the source of nitrogen |
|---|---|
| Uridine 5'-monophosphate (UMP) can be converted into what compound? | Cytidine monophosphate (CMP) |
| What is the difference between UMP and TMP? | TMP is the methylated version of UMP |
| Can the unmodified products of purine and pyrimidine synthesis be used for RNA synthesis? | Yes |
| Can the unmodified products of purine and pyrimidine synthesis be used for DNA synthesis? | No, they must be converted from ribonucleotides to deoxyribonucleotides |
| What enzyme catalyzes the conversion of ribonucleotides to deoxyribonucleotides? | Ribonucleotide reductase |
| What molecule inhibits this enzyme? | dATP |

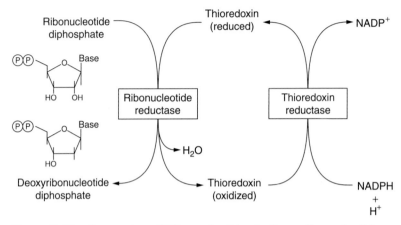

**Figure 2.15** Conversion of Ribonucleotides to Deoxyribonucleotides.

## AMINO ACID TRANSPORT

| | |
|---|---|
| **What is the first step in the breakdown of amino acids?** | Removal of the $\alpha$-amino group, usually transferring this group to $\alpha$-ketogluatarate |
| **What enzymes participate in the transfer of $\alpha$-amino groups?** | ALT and AST |
| **Elevations in the plasma levels of the aforementioned enzymes are correlated with disease in what organ?** | Liver |
| **What step follows glutamate formation?** | Oxidative deamination of glutamate |
| **What enzyme catalyzes this reaction?** | Glutamate dehydrogenase |
| **What coenzymes does this enzyme utilize?** | $NAD^+$ and $NADP^+$ |

## UREA CYCLE

| | |
|---|---|
| **What is the function of urea?** | To dispose of amino groups from amino acids, because ammonia is toxic to the body (particularly the central nervous system [CNS]) |
| **What molecules provide the two nitrogen atoms of urea?** | One nitrogen comes from free $NH_3$ and the other nitrogen comes from aspartate (the carbon and oxygen of urea comes from $CO_2$) |

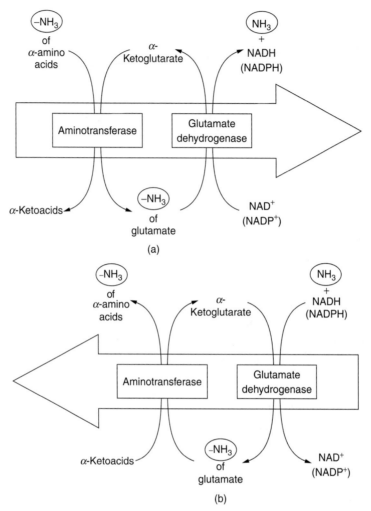

**Figure 2.16**  Disposal and Synthesis of Amino Acids. (a) Disposal; (b) Synthesis.

| | |
|---|---|
| **Where in the body does the urea cycle take place?** | Liver |
| **Where in the cell does the urea cycle take place?** | The first two reactions take place in the mitochondria and the rest of the cycle takes place in the cytosol |
| **What two molecules are able to cross the mitochondrial membrane?** | Ornithine and citrulline |
| **What is the rate-limiting step of the urea cycle?** | Formation of carbamoyl phosphate |

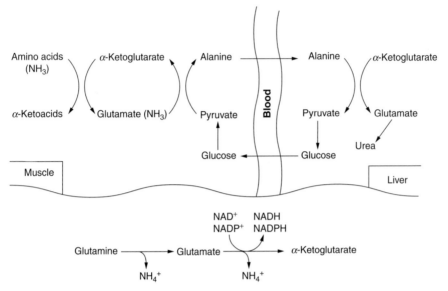

**Figure 2.17** Ammonium Transport by Alanine and Glutamine.

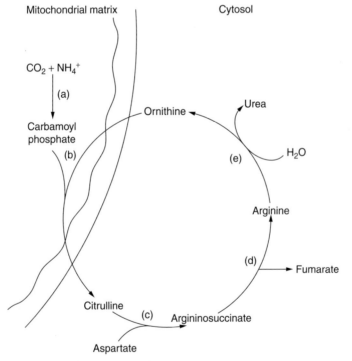

**Figure 2.18** Urea Cycle. (a) Carbamoyl Phosphate Synthase; (b) Ornithine Transcarbamoylase; (c) Argininosuccinate Synthase; (d) Aminotransferase; (e) Arginase.

| | |
|---|---|
| What enzyme catalyzes the rate-limiting step of the urea cycle? | CPS I |
| How many phosphate groups are used in the formation of urea? | Four |
| Where in the body is urea transported for excretion? | Kidneys |

## CHOLESTEROL, LIPOPROTEINS, AND STEROID BIOSYNTHESIS

| | |
|---|---|
| What molecule provides the carbon pool for steroid synthesis? | Acetate |
| What organ plays the most significant role in cholesterol balance? | Liver |
| Which molecule provides the reducing equivalents for cholesterol synthesis? | NADPH |
| What enzyme catalyzes the rate-limiting step in the synthesis of cholesterol? | Hydroxymethylglutaryl (HMG)-CoA reductase |
| What series of reactions make the synthesis of cholesterol essentially irreversible? | The four condensation reactions which release pyrophosphate |
| Which molecules provide feedback inhibition to HMG-CoA reductase? | Cholesterol, cAMP |
| Name a hormone which decreases the rate of cholesterol synthesis. | Glucagon |
| How does this type of negative regulation occur? | Glucagon favors formation of the phosphorylated (inactive) form of HMG-CoA reductase |
| Name a hormone which increases the rate of cholesterol synthesis. | Insulin |
| How does this type of negative regulation occur? | Insulin favors the formation of the unphosphorylated (active) form of HMG-CoA reductase |
| How do sterols inhibit de novo cholesterol synthesis? | Chylomicrons remnants and low-density lipoproteins (LDLs) taken up by the liver decrease the genetic transcription of HMG-CoA reductase |
| Name three organs that convert cholesterol into steroid hormones. | Adrenal cortex |
| | Gonads (testes and ovaries) |
| | Placenta |

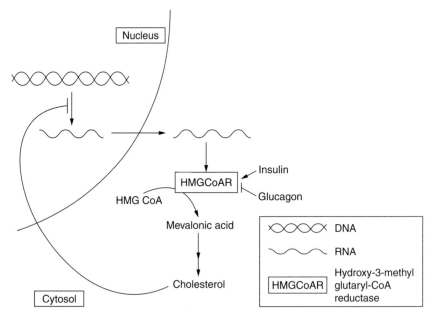

**Figure 2.19    HMG CoA Regulation.**

| | |
|---|---|
| **What is the mechanism of action of statins?** | Inhibit HMG-CoA reductase and decrease the rate of de novo cholesterol synthesis |
| **What is the composition of a lipoprotein?** | Varying proportions of cholesterol, triglycerides, and phospholipids in addition to associated apolipoproteins |
| **Name the four major apolipoproteins and list their functions.** | A-I activates lechitin-cholesterol acyltransferase |
| | B-100 binds the LDL receptor |
| | C-II cofactor for lipoprotein lipase |
| | E mediates excess remnant uptake |
| **What is the function of a chylomicron?** | To deliver triglycerides to peripheral tissues and dietary cholesterol to the liver |
| **What cells make chylomicrons?** | Enterocytes |
| **What is the function of very low-density lipoproteins (VLDLs)?** | To deliver hepatic triglycerides to peripheral tissues |
| **Where are VLDLs secreted from?** | Liver |
| **What is the function of LDLs?** | To deliver hepatic cholesterol to peripheral tissues |

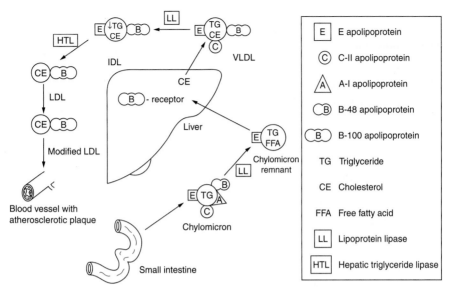

**Figure 2.20**   Lipoprotein Metabolism.

| | |
|---|---|
| **How are LDLs formed?** | Via the modification of VLDLs by lipoprotein lipase in peripheral tissues |
| **How are LDLs taken up into target cells?** | Receptor-mediated endocytosis |
| **What is the pathophysiology behind familial hypercholesterolemia?** | Increased LDL (bad cholesterol) due to a defective LDL receptor |
| **What total cholesterol level can be found in individuals heterozygous for the aforementioned mutation?** | About 300 mg/dL |
| **What total cholesterol level can be found in individuals homozygous for the aforementioned mutation?** | About 700 mg/dL |
| **What are the symptoms of familial hypercholesterolemia type IIa?** | Severe atherosclerosis early in life, possible myocardial infarction before 20 years of age, xanthomas |
| **Familial hypercholesterolemia type IIa is inherited in what pattern?** | Autosomal dominant |
| **Where are high-density lipoproteins (HDLs) secreted from?** | Liver and intestine |
| **What is the function of an HDL?** | To mediate transport of cholesterol from peripheral tissues to the liver |

| | |
|---|---|
| **Intermediate density lipoproteins (IDLs) are formed from the degradation of what lipoproteins?** | VLDLs |
| **What is the function of an IDL?** | To deliver triglycerides and cholesterol to the liver |
| **What is the structure of triglycerides?** | Three fatty acids esterified to a glycerol backbone |
| **What enzyme hydrolyzes triglycerides?** | Lipase |
| **What substance secreted by the liver aids in the digestion of fatty acids?** | Bile |
| **Where is bile stored?** | Gall bladder |
| **Bile duct obstruction can lead to a deficiency in what vitamins?** | Vitamins A, D, E, and K |
| **Why does bile duct obstruction lead to this deficiency?** | Absorption of these vitamins is dependent on the presence of bile |
| **Following the absorption of triglycerides by the epithelial cells of the small intestine, what are triglycerides combined to form?** | Chylomicrons |
| **What must happen to a chylomicron in order for it to be taken up by tissue?** | Hydrolysis by clearing factor lipase (i.e., lipoprotein lipase) |
| **Lipoprotein lipase hydrolyzes chylomicrons into what molecules?** | 2-Monoacylglycerol and fatty acids |
| **Triglyceride is transported from the liver to adipose tissue in what form?** | VLDL |
| **What enzyme is activated in the fasted state to mobilize stored triglycerides?** | Hormone-sensitive lipase |
| **Name the four principal functions of fatty acids.** | Components of phospholipids |
| | Lipophilic modifiers of proteins |
| | Fuel molecules |
| | Hormones and intracellular messengers |
| **Name two types of cells which cannot utilize fatty acids as a form of energy.** | Erythrocytes and brain cells |
| **What molecule, which can replace glucose as a fuel, can fatty acids be converted into?** | Ketone bodies |
| **Glycerol is utilized by what tissue?** | Liver |
| **What is glycerol converted to in this tissue?** | Dihydroxyacetone phosphate (i.e., DHAP, which can be converted to glucose) |

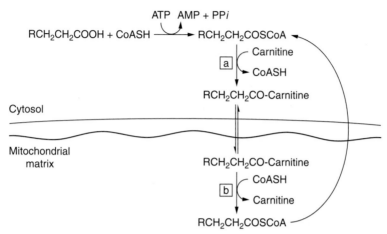

**Figure 2.21** Fatty Acid Transport. (a) Carnitine acyltransferase I; (b) Carnitine acyltransferase II.

| | |
|---|---|
| What two enzymes transport fatty acids across the mitochondrial membrane? | Carnitine palmitoyltransferases (I and II) |
| Defects in the carnitine transport system can lead to what clinical manifestations? | Hypoglycemia, muscle wasting |
| What is the name of the process that oxidizes fatty acids to acetyl CoA? | $\beta$-Oxidation |
| Where in the cell does this process occur? | Mitochondrial matrix |
| How does malonyl CoA inhibit the oxidation of fatty acids? | Inhibits carnitine palmitoyltransferase I |
| What is the final product of fatty acid oxidation? | Propionyl CoA |
| This product must be converted into what molecule in order to enter the TCA cycle? | Succinyl CoA |
| What reaction does propionyl-CoA carboxylase catalyze? | Propionyl CoA to methylmalonyl CoA |
| What is the pathophysiology behind propionyl-CoA carboxylase deficiency? | Deficiency of propionyl-CoA carboxylase causes odd-numbered fatty acid chains to build up and accumulate in the liver |
| What are the symptoms of propionyl-CoA carboxylase deficiency? | Episodic lethargy, anorexia, vomiting, acidosis, CNS depression, and developmental problems |
| What inheritance pattern is seen in propionyl-CoA carboxylase deficiency? | Autosomal recessive |

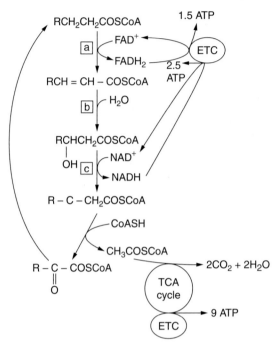

**Figure 2.22** Pathway for β-Oxidation. (a) Acyl-CoA dehydrogenase; (b) Enoyl Hydratase; (c) β-Hydroxyacyl-CoA dehydrogenase.

| | |
|---|---|
| Name the ketone bodies. | Acetoacetate, β-hydroxybutyrate, acetone |
| What two characteristics of ketone bodies make them a good fuel for the glucose-starved brain? | Free solubility in blood, easy crossing of the blood-brain barrier |
| What two tissues synthesize fatty acids? | Adipose tissue and liver |
| Where in the cell does fatty acid synthesis occur? | Cytosol |
| What is the principal regulated reaction in fatty acid synthesis? | Acetyl CoA + $CO_2$ + ATP → malonyl CoA + ADP + $P_i$ |
| What enzyme catalyzes this reaction? | Acetyl-CoA carboxylase |
| What are the main hormone regulators of this enzyme? | Stimulated by insulin; inhibited by glucagon and epinephrine |
| Name two allosteric regulators of this enzyme. | Citrate (+), palmitoyl CoA (−) |

# CHAPTER 3

# Nutrition

## ENERGY NEEDS

| | |
|---|---|
| What is the basal energy expenditure? | Energy used for metabolic processes while at rest |
| The basal energy expenditure represents what percentage of the total energy expenditure? | 60% |
| What is the thermic effect of food? | Energy required for digesting and absorbing food |
| The thermic effect of food represents what percentage of the total energy expenditure? | 10% |
| What is the activity-related expenditure? | Energy that varies with the level of physical activity |
| The activity-related expenditure represents what percentage of the total energy expenditure? | 20–30% |
| What is the estimated daily energy need for an infant? | 120 kcal/kg dry body weight |
| What is the estimated daily energy need for an adult? | 30 kcal/kg dry body weight |
| What is the caloric yield from 1 g of carbohydrate? | 4 kcal |
| What is the caloric yield from 1 g of protein? | 4 kcal |
| What is the caloric yield from 1 g of fat? | 9 kcal |
| What is the caloric yield from 1 g of alcohol? | 7 kcal |

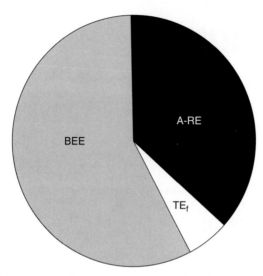

**Figure 3.1**  Total Energy Expenditure. BEE—Basal energy expenditure,
TE$_f$—Thermic effect of food, A–RE—Activity-related expenditure.

## MACRONUTRIENTS

| | |
|---|---|
| **Carbohydrates should typically comprise what percentage of the total caloric intake?** | 50–60% |
| **What is the difference between "available" and "unavailable" carbohydrates?** | "Available" carbohydrates can be used by tissues for fuel; "unavailable" carbohydrates are not digested or absorbed but do provide bulk to the diet and assist in elimination. |
| **List the "available" carbohydrates.** | Glucose, fructose, sucrose, lactose, maltose, starches, dextrins, glycogen |
| **List the "unavailable" carbohydrates.** | Cellulose, hemicellulose, lignin, pectins, gums |
| **Inadequate carbohydrate intake may lead to what catastrophic processes?** | Ketosis, wasting, cationic loss, dehydration |
| **In what forms are excess carbohydrates stored in the body?** | Glycogen, triacylglycerol |
| **Fats should typically comprise what percentage of the total caloric intake?** | 30% (saturated fats should make up less than 10%) |
| **List the essential fatty acids.** | Linoleic acid, linolenic acid |

| | |
|---|---|
| **What functions do fats have in the body?** | Precursors for synthesis of prostaglandins, prostacyclins, leukotrienes, and thromboxanes; carriers of fat-soluble vitamins; slow gastric emptying; give foods a desirable texture and taste |
| **What characteristic symptom is associated with inadequate fat intake?** | Scaly dermatitis |
| **In what form is excess fat stored in the body?** | Triacylglycerol |
| **Proteins should typically comprise what percentage of the total caloric intake?** | 10–20% |
| **What is the recommended adult protein intake?** | 0.8 g/kg body weight per day |
| **List the nine essential amino acids that cannot be synthesized in the body from nonprotein precursors.** | PVT TIM H*LL (i.e., phenylalanine, valine, tryptophan, threonine, isoleucine, methionine, histidine, leucine, lysine) |
| **What function do proteins have in the body?** | Provide amino acids for synthesizing proteins and nonprotein nitrogenous bases |
| **What is nitrogen balance?** | The difference between nitrogen intake (protein) and nitrogen excretion (undigested protein in the feces + urea in the urine + ammonia in the urine) |
| **In what instances would an individual be in positive nitrogen balance?** | Pregnancy/lactation, growth, recovery from trauma/infection/surgery |
| **In what instances would an individual be in negative nitrogen balance?** | Metabolic stress, insufficient dietary protein, insufficient intake of an essential amino acid |
| **What is kwashiorkor?** | A form of malnutrition caused by inadequate protein intake in the presence of adequate total caloric intake (often occurs in areas of limited food/protein supply and/or inadequate knowledge of proper diet) |
| **What are the clinical features of kwashiorkor?** | Fatigue, irritability, growth failure, loss of muscle mass, protuberant belly, edema; skin disorders such as vitiligo, alopecia, and dermatitis are also common; severe, late stage protein deficiency can lead to shock, coma, or death |

| | |
|---|---|
| **What is marasmus?** | Protein-energy malnutrition that results from a negative energy balance (decreased total caloric intake, increased energy expenditure, or a combination of both) |
| **What are the clinical features of marasmus?** | Children adapt to the energy deficit with a decrease in physical activity, lethargy, slowing of growth, and weight loss; other clinical features include anemia, edema, tachypnea, and abdominal distention |
| **What equation calculates BMI (body mass index)?** | Weight (kg)/Height (m$^2$) = BMI (kg/m$^2$) |
| **What is an ideal BMI?** | 19–25 |
| **What BMI is correlated with obesity for women? For men?** | Over 32; over 31 |
| **What is the correlation between BMI and poor health?** | The risk of poor health increases with increasing BMI |
| **List the diseases associated with obesity.** | Coronary artery disease, hypertension, non-insulin-dependent diabetes mellitus, breast and uterine cancer, gallstone formation, osteoarthritis, respiratory problems |

## WATER-SOLUBLE VITAMINS

| | |
|---|---|
| **Name the water-soluble vitamins.** | B-complex vitamins (B$_1$, B$_2$, B$_3$, B$_5$, B$_6$, B$_{12}$), folate, vitamin C, and biotin |
| **What is the physiological function of vitamin B$_1$ (thiamine)?** | Cofactor in the hexose monophosphate (HMP) shunt and in the oxidative decarboxylation of $\alpha$-ketoacids (i.e., pyruvate, $\alpha$-ketoglutarate) |
| **What is the RDA (recommended dietary allowance) of vitamin B$_1$?** | 1 mg |
| **Which two clinical syndromes are associated with thiamine deficiency, particularly in alcoholics?** | Beriberi and Wernicke-Korsakoff syndrome |
| **What are the clinical features of beriberi syndrome?** | Polyneuritis *(dry)*, dilated cardiomyopathy *(wet)*, and edema |
| **What are the clinical features of Wernicke-Korsakoff syndrome?** | Gait disturbance, diplopia, confabulation, and memory loss |

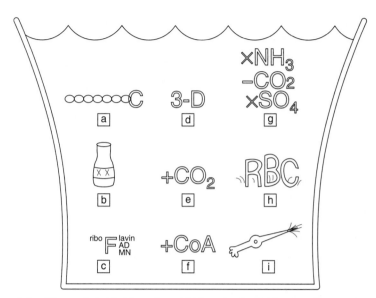

**Figure 3.2** Water-Soluble Vitamins. (a) Vitamin C; (b) Vitamin $B_1$; (c) Vitamin $B_2$; (d) Vitamin $B_3$; (e) Biotin; (f) Vitamin $B_5$; (g) Vitamin $B_6$; (h) Folate; (i) Vitamin $B_{12}$.

| | |
|---|---|
| Name two pathways that utilize folate as a cofactor. | Purine and pyrimidine synthesis |
| What is the RDA of folate? | 400 µg |
| What are the two most common causes of folate deficiency? | Pregnancy and alcoholism |
| What is the danger associated with folate deficiency during pregnancy? | Neural tube defects (i.e., spina bifida, anencephaly) |
| What characteristic features are found on a peripheral blood smear in patients with folate deficiency? | Megaloblastic (macrocytic) anemia |
| Name three medications that can interfere with folate utilization in the body. | Dilantin, phenytoin (anticonvulsants), methotrexate (cancer and rheumatoid arthritis), sulfasalazine (Crohn's disease and ulcerative colitis), trimethoprim (antibacterial), pyrimethamine (antimalarial) |
| What is the mechanism of action of sulfonamide antibiotics? | Sulfonamide antibiotics mimic p-aminobenzoic acid (PABA), a folate precursor, competing with the physiological precursor for the enzyme involved in the next step of folate synthesis |

| | |
|---|---|
| **Which vitamin is a cofactor in both gluconeogenesis and fatty acid synthesis?** | Biotin |
| **Name three reactions that use biotin as a cofactor.** | Carboxylations of pyruvate to oxaloacetate, acetyl coenzyme A (CoA) to malonyl CoA, and propionyl CoA to methylmalonyl CoA |
| **What is the RDA of biotin?** | 30 μg/day |
| **Name some clinical features of biotin deficiency.** | Hair loss, bowel inflammation, muscle pain, dermatitis |
| **What vitamin deficiency is associated with the excessive consumption of raw eggs?** | Biotin deficiency (avidin strongly binds biotin) |
| **Which coenzymes are derived from vitamin $B_3$ (niacin) and in which types of reactions are these coenzymes used?** | Nicotinamide adenine dinucleotide, NAD(H) and nicotine adenine dinucleotide phosphate, NADP(H); used in oxidation/reduction reactions |
| **What is the RDA of niacin?** | 14–16 mg |
| **What clinical features are typically associated with pellagra?** | Dementia, dermatitis, diarrhea (death, if untreated) |
| **Name three common causes of niacin deficiency.** | Isoniazid (INH) treatment, Hartnup disease (autosomal dominant disease with impaired transport of neutral amino acids in the kidneys and small intestine), and malignant carcinoid syndrome |
| **What coenzymes are derived from vitamin $B_2$ (riboflavin)?** | Flavin adenine dinucleotide, $FAD^+$ ($FADH_2$) |
| **What is the RDA of riboflavin?** | 1.1–1.3 mg |
| **What clinical features are commonly associated with vitamin $B_2$ (riboflavin) deficiency?** | Corneal neovascularization, cheliosis/stomatitis, and magenta-colored tongue |
| **Vitamin $B_5$ (pantothenate) is used as a precursor in which coenzyme?** | CoA |
| **What is considered adequate intake of pantothenate?** | 5 mg/day |
| **What are the common clinical features of pantothenate deficiency?** | Adrenal insufficiency, enteritis, dermatitis, and hair loss |
| **How is vitamin $B_6$ (pyridoxine) activated in the body?** | Pyridoxine is converted into pyridoxal phosphate |

| | |
|---|---|
| Which enzymes make use of this active form? | Aminotransferase (aspartate aminotransferase, alanine aminotransferase [AST, ALT]), decarboxylation, and transsulfuration enzymes |
| What is the RDA of vitamin $B_6$? | 1.1–1.7 mg |
| What are the clinical features of vitamin $B_6$ deficiency? | Convulsions, hyperirritability, cheliosis/stomatitis, and sideroblastic anemia |
| Name two drugs that can induce a deficiency of vitamin $B_6$. | INH and oral contraceptives |
| High doses of vitamin $B_6$ may be used to treat what disease? | Homocystinuria |
| How is vitamin $B_{12}$ (cobalamin) synthesized, absorbed, and stored by the body? | Synthesized by microorganisms in the small intestine, absorbed by an intrinsic-factor mediated mechanism in the terminal ileum, and stored in the liver |
| What is the RDA of vitamin $B_{12}$? | 2.4 µg/day |
| What are some dietary sources of vitamin $B_{12}$? | Animal products including eggs, meat, and dairy |
| Name two enzymes that require $B_{12}$ as a cofactor. | Homocysteine methyltransferase in homocysteine methylation and methylmalonyl CoA mutase in methylmalonyl CoA processing |
| List some causes of vitamin $B_{12}$ deficiency. | Celiac disease, enteritis, *Diphyllobothrium latum* infection (tapeworm), alcoholism, Crohn's disease, strict vegan/vegetarian diet, gastrectomy, terminal ileum resection, or bacterial overgrowth in the small intestine (deficiency is usually due to malabsorption, not insufficient dietary supply) |
| What is the pathophysiology of pernicious anemia? | Deficiency of intrinsic factor in gastric secretions (may be caused by antiparietal cell antibodies) resulting in decreased vitamin $B_{12}$ absorption |
| What are two common clinical consequences of vitamin $B_{12}$ deficiency? | Megaloblastic (macrocytic) anemia and progressive peripheral neuropathy |

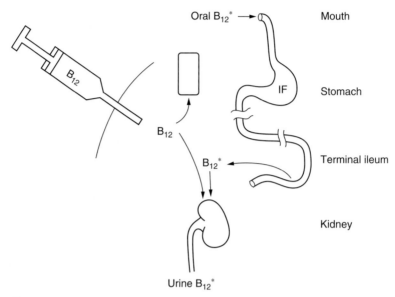

**Figure 3.3**   Schilling Test.

**What laboratory test can help uncover the cause of low serum $B_{12}$ levels?**

Schilling test: In Part I, radio-labeled vitamin $B_{12}$ is given by mouth and a large dose of unlabeled vitamin $B_{12}$ is given by intramuscular (IM) injection to saturate cellular uptake mechanisms. If the amount of label appearing in the urine over 24 hours is low, due to decreased gut absorption, then Part II tests whether any identified malabsorption of vitamin $B_{12}$ is due to a lack of intrinsic factor by giving exogenous intrinsic factor in a repeat test.

**Name three medications that can decrease levels of vitamin $B_{12}$.**

Metformin, phenytoin, and methotrexate

**Name three physiological roles of vitamin C (ascorbic acid).**

Hydroxylation of proline and lysine residues in collagen synthesis, facilitation of iron absorption in the gastrointestinal (GI) tract by maintaining iron in the more absorbable reduced state ($Fe^{2+}$), and as a cofactor utilized in the conversion of dopamine to norepinephrine

| | |
|---|---|
| **What are some dietary sources of vitamin C?** | Citrus fruits and green vegetables (deficiency is associated with a diet low in these sources) |
| **What is the RDA of vitamin C?** | 75–90 mg |
| **Name some clinical features of vitamin C deficiency (scurvy).** | Poor wound healing, easy bruising, bleeding gums, glossitis, and increased bleeding time |

## FAT-SOLUBLE VITAMINS

| | |
|---|---|
| **Which vitamins are dependent upon lipid emulsification for absorption?** | The fat-soluble vitamins (vitamins A, D, E, and K) |
| **Name some conditions that can cause a deficiency of fat-soluble vitamins.** | Tropical or celiac sprue, cystic fibrosis, chronic pancreatitis, lactose intolerance, extended antibiotic use, and excessive mineral oil intake |
| **Do water-soluble or fat-soluble vitamins more often cause toxicity? Why?** | Fat-soluble vitamins, because they accumulate in fat |
| **How is vitamin D synthesized by the body?** | 7-Dehydrocholesterol, derived from cholesterol, is synthesized in the liver; UV rays on sun-exposed skin convert 7-dehydrocholesterol into cholecal-ciferol (the storage form of vitamin D) |

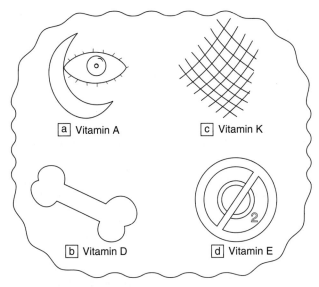

**Figure 3.4**   Fat-Soluble Vitamins.

| | |
|---|---|
| **Name one dietary source of vitamin D.** | Commercial dairy products (contain UV-irradiated ergocalciferol derived from yeast) |
| **What is considered adequate intake of vitamin D?** | 5 µg/day |
| **How is vitamin D (cholecalciferol) converted to its active form?** | Stored cholecalciferol in the liver is hydroxylated to 25-hydroxycholecalciferol by liver enzymes; when serum calcium is low, the parathyroid gland releases parathyroid hormone (PTH) which activates $1\alpha$-hydroxylase to convert 25-hydroxycholecalciferol to 1,25-dihydroxycholecalciferol (1,25-DHCC) in a second hydroxylation. |
| **What is the role of active 1,25-DHCC in calcium homeostasis?** | Increases intestinal calcium uptake by acting as a lipid-soluble hormone on duodenal epithelia and increases calcium reabsorption in the kidney; 1,25-DHCC also acts in conjunction with PTH to mobilize the calcium stores found in bone |
| **Name three medical conditions that decrease vitamin D activity.** | End-stage renal disease (resulting in decreased $1\alpha$-hydroxylase activity in proximal tubule cells), Fanconi syndrome (a defect in proximal renal tubule cells), and genetic deficiency of the $1\alpha$-hydroxylase enzyme (vitamin D-resistant rickets) |
| **What condition is the result of vitamin D deficiency during childhood?** | Rickets |
| **What are the clinical features of this disorder?** | Skeletal abnormalities (bowing deformities of the legs and other developing bones), osteomalacia (bone softening due to vitamin D deficiency following epiphyseal closure) |
| **What symptoms do you expect to find with hypercalcemia?** | Stupor, change in mental status, nausea/vomiting, flank pain, and polyuria |
| **Which drugs can cause hypercalcemia when taken along with vitamin D and/or related compounds?** | Thiazide diuretics (decrease calcium excretion in the kidney) |
| **What is the role of vitamin A in epithelial cells?** | Growth, differentiation, and maintenance |

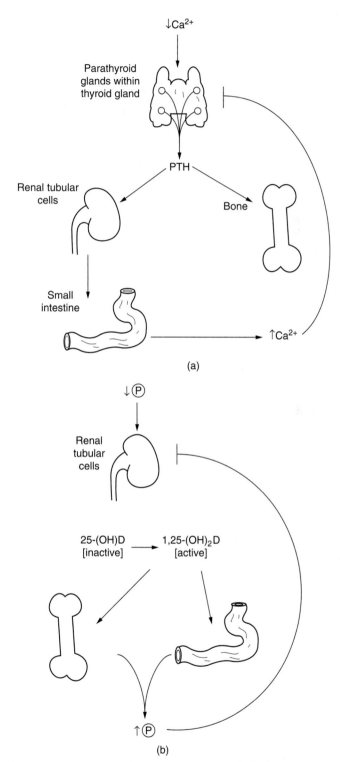

**Figure 3.5** Calcium Homeostasis. (a) PTH Regulation; (b) Vitamin D Regulation.

**What is the role of vitamin A in visual pigments?**

Converted into cis-retinal and acts as a cofactor for opsin (protein that synthesizes rhodopsin which is utilized in rods for night vision)

**What is the role of vitamin A in the immune system?**

Maintenance of mucous membranes, plays a role in leukocyte function

**What is the RDA of vitamin A?**

700–900 µg retinol activity equivalents per day

**Name some potential signs of vitamin A deficiency.**

Night blindness, dry eyes, dry skin, bronchitis, pneumonia, and impaired immune response

**Name some consequences of vitamin A excess.**

Arthralgia, headaches, fatigue, skin changes, sore throat, and hair loss

**What is the major physiological role of vitamin E?**

Antioxidant; also counteracts atherosclerotic changes and coronary artery disease by preventing the oxidation of low-density lipoprotein (LDL) particles

**What is the RDA of vitamin E?**

15 mg

**List the dietary sources of vitamin E.**

Green leafy vegetables and seed grains

**What is the most significant feature of vitamin E deficiency?**

Erythrocytes will demonstrate increased osmotic and peroxidative fragility, causing hemolytic anemia

**Name a test which can be used to help diagnose vitamin E deficiency.**

Osmotic fragility test (also used to test for hereditary spherocytosis)

**What is the most significant source of vitamin K in a healthy person?**

Synthesis by intestinal bacteria

**What is the physiological role of vitamin K?**

$\gamma$-Carboxylation of the coagulation factors II, VII, IX, X and proteins C and S

**What is considered adequate intake of vitamin K?**

90–120 µg

**Name some causes of vitamin K deficiency.**

Fat malabsorption syndromes, long-term antibiotic therapy (removes intestinal flora), breast-feeding infants (lack intestinal flora), anticonvulsant drugs (i.e., phenyldantoins)

| | |
|---|---|
| **What are the clinical features of vitamin K deficiency?** | Mild vitamin K deficiency will prolong prothrombin time (PT), but partial thromboplastin time (PTT) will be normal; in neonates, vitamin K deficiency will cause hemorrhage with increased PT and activated partial thromboplastin time (aPTT), but normal bleeding time; severe vitamin K deficiency will prolong PT and PTT |
| **What are the clinical features of vitamin K toxicity in infants?** | Anemia, hyperbilirubinemia, kernicterus |
| **Name a drug which antagonizes the physiological activity of vitamin K.** | Warfarin (Coumadin) |

## MINERALS

| | |
|---|---|
| **What bodily functions require calcium?** | Formation of bones and teeth, nerve and muscle function, blood clotting |
| **What are the dietary sources of calcium?** | Dairy products, leafy green vegetables, fortified foods |
| **What is the RDA of calcium?** | 1000 mg |
| **What are the signs and symptoms of calcium deficiency?** | Paresthesias, increased neuromuscular excitability, muscle cramps, bone fractures, osteomalacia |
| **Iodine is required for the formation of what biologically important hormone?** | Thyroid hormone |
| **What are the dietary sources of iodine?** | Seafood (i.e., shellfish), iodized salt |
| **What is the RDA of iodine?** | 150 mg |
| **What are the signs and symptoms of iodine deficiency?** | Goiter, cretinism |
| **Iron is utilized by what biologically important molecules?** | Hemoglobin, myoglobin, cytochromes, oxidases, oxygenases |
| **What foods have high iron content?** | Liver, heart, wheat germ, egg yolks, oysters, fruits, dried beans |
| **What is the RDA of iron in adult men? Adult women?** | 8 mg in adult men; 18 mg in adult women |
| **Where in the GI tract is iron absorbed?** | Duodenum |
| **Is heme iron or nonheme iron absorbed more efficiently?** | Heme iron |

| | |
|---|---|
| **What substances enhance iron absorption?** | Vitamin C, reducing sugars, meat |
| **What substances reduce iron absorption?** | Antacids, fiber, oxalate |
| **What are the signs and symptoms of iron deficiency?** | Hypochromic microcytic anemia, fatigue, pallor, tachycardia, shortness of breath on exertion, depapillation of the tongue, pica |
| **What is hemochromatosis?** | Iron toxicity with increased deposition of iron in many organs |
| **What is the classic triad of hemochromatosis?** | Micronodular pigment cirrhosis, *bronze* diabetes, skin pigmentation |
| **What stain is used histologically to diagnose hemochromatosis?** | Prussian blue |
| **Hemochromatosis can predispose an individual to what diseases?** | Congestive heart failure, hepatocellular carcinoma |
| **What is the treatment for hemochromatosis?** | Repeated phlebotomy, IV deferoxamine |
| **What are the physiological roles of magnesium in the body?** | Binding to the active site of enzymes, complexing with adenosine triphosphate (ATP) |
| **List the richest dietary sources of magnesium.** | Dairy products, grains, nuts |
| **What is the RDA of magnesium?** | 320–420 mg |
| **Magnesium deficiency is often seen in individuals with what concurrent disorders?** | Alcoholism, fat malabsorption syndromes, hypocalcemia |
| **What are the signs and symptoms of magnesium deficiency?** | Increased neuromuscular excitability, depression of PTH release (with severe hypomagnesemia) leading to hypocalcemia |
| **Describe the roles of phosphorous (phosphate) in the body.** | Structural when found in bone or DNA/RNA, buffer when found in blood, energy storage when found in ATP, compartmentalizing when found in plasma membranes |
| **What dietary sources are rich in phosphorous?** | Seafood, nuts, grains, legumes, cheese |
| **What is the RDA of phosphorous?** | 700 mg |
| **What is the most common cause of phosphorous deficiency?** | Renal failure |

| | |
|---|---|
| **What are the signs and symptoms of phosphorous deficiency?** | Defective bone mineralization with retarded growth, skeletal deformities, bone pain, decreased 2,3-bisphosphoglycerate leading to tissue hypoxia |
| **Zinc is required for the function of what physiologically important molecules?** | Metalloenzymes |
| **What dietary sources are rich in zinc?** | Meat, eggs, seafood, whole grains |
| **What is the RDA of zinc?** | 8–11 mg |
| **What are the signs and symptoms of zinc deficiency?** | Growth retardation, hypogonadism, impaired taste and smell, poor appetite, reduced immune function, mental lethargy, dry and scaly skin |
| **What are the signs and symptoms of zinc toxicity?** | Vomiting, diarrhea; neurological damage upon inhalation of zinc oxide fumes |

# CHAPTER 4

# Molecular Biology

## OVERVIEW

| | |
|---|---|
| **What constitutes a nucleoside?** | A nitrogenous base linked to a pentose monosaccharide |
| **What constitutes a nucleotide?** | A nitrogenous base, a pentose monosaccharide, and either 1, 2, or 3 phosphate groups (basically a phosphorylated nucleoside) |
| **Which constituent(s) carries genetic information?** | The nitrogenous base |
| **Which constituent(s) maintains the backbone of DNA?** | The sugar and phosphate groups |
| **Name the two families of nitrogenous bases.** | Purines and pyrimidines |
| **What is the difference between a purine and a pyrimidine?** | Purines contain two rings whereas pyrimidines contain one ring |
| **Name the two bases in the purine class.** | Adenine and guanine (remember PURE As Gold) |
| **Name the three bases in the pyrimidine class.** | Cytosine, uracil, and thymine (remember PYRAMIDS are CUT) |
| **How do uracil and thymine differ in structure?** | Thymine contains a methyl group (THYmine contains meTHYl) |
| **What bases can be found in DNA?** | Adenine, guanine, thymine, and cytosine |
| **What bases can be found in RNA?** | Adenine, guanine, uracil, and cytosine |
| **Describe the polarity of the DNA chain.** | One end of the chain has a 5'-OH group and the other a 3'-OH group; therefore, the base sequence is written in the 5' $\rightarrow$ 3' direction |

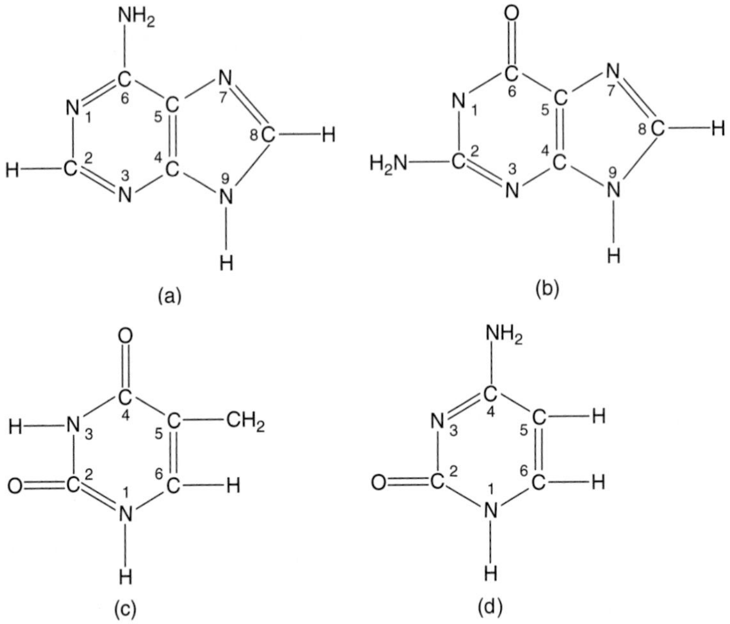

**Figure 4.1** Nitrogenous Bases. (a) Adenine; (b) Guanine;
(c) Thymine; (d) Cytosine.

**What bases pair with each other in the complementary strands of DNA?**

Adenine pairs with thymine (held together by two hydrogen bonds), guanine pairs with cytosine (held together by three hydrogen bonds); the guanine-cytosine base pair has a stronger bond

**List the important features of the Watson and Crick model of DNA.**

Double helix, with the sugar-phosphate chains running in opposite directions

Base pairs are on the inside of the double helix

Helical structure repeats after 10 residues on each chain; helix turns 360° every 10 residues

Chains are held together via hydrogen bonding between bases

Genetic information is carried in the precise sequence of bases

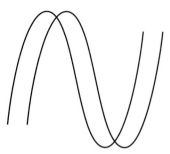

**Figure 4.2** DNA Double Helix.

What are some key differences between DNA and RNA?

DNA is usually double-stranded (in a double-helix format), RNA is usually single-stranded; the sugar in DNA is deoxyribose, the sugar in RNA is ribose; DNA utilizes adenine, thymine, guanine, and cytosine as bases, RNA utilizes adenine, uracil, guanine, and cytosine as bases

What are the two stages of making proteins?

Transcription (DNA to RNA) and translation (RNA to protein)

In what direction is DNA replicated?

$5'$ to $3'$

What are plasmids?

Small, circular, extrachromosomal DNA molecules that may or may not be synchronized with chromosomal division

What type of information can be carried by a plasmid?

The genes for inactivation of antibiotics, production of toxins, and/or breakdown of natural products

What is the importance of plasmids in pharmacology?

Plasmids may be used by microorganisms to confer resistance to a specific antibiotic

## LABORATORY TECHNIQUES

What separation methods can be used to yield a purified protein based upon:

Size?

Gel filtration, preparative gel electrophoresis

Ionic charge?

Gel electrophoresis, ion-exchange chromatography

Binding to ligands or antibodies?

Affinity chromatography

|  |  |
|---|---|
| List chemicals/enzymes used to selectively cleave proteins. | Trypsin, chymotrypsin, 2-nitro-5-thiocyanobenzene, cyanogen bromide |
| Enzyme-linked immunosorbent assay (ELISA) tests what type of reactivity? | Antigen-antibody reactivity (an antibody test to an exposed antigen) |
| When is ELISA used? | In the serodiagnosis of specific infectious diseases (i.e., human immunodeficiency virus [HIV]) to determine whether a particular antibody is present in a patient's blood sample |
| What methods are used to determine the three-dimensional structure of a protein? | X-ray crystallography, nuclear magnetic resonance |
| Describe the action of a restriction endonuclease. | Recognizes specific base sequences (typically palindromic sequences) in double-helical DNA and cleaves both strands of the duplex at specific sites |
| How is the action of a restriction endonuclease of benefit in gel electrophoresis? | Small differences in base sequence between related DNA molecules result in different sized restriction fragments upon exposure to a restriction endonuclease; gel electrophoresis is then used to separate these fragments based on molecular size |
| What is the relationship between the thickness of a band on an electrophoresis gel and the abundance of restriction fragment? | Thickness of the band is directly proportional to the abundance of restriction fragment |
| What probe is used in Southern blotting? | Labeled DNA probe |
| What probe is used in Northern blotting? | Labeled RNA probe |
| What is a Western blot? | Separation of proteins via electrophoresis followed by identification by specific complexing with antibodies that are tagged with a radio-labeled second protein |
| What is the Sanger dideoxynucleotide method used to determine? | The sequence of bases in DNA fragments |
| List the steps of the Sanger dideoxynucleotide method. | Denature the DNA fragment into single strands and divide them into four samples |

Add the following to each sample: an oligonucleotide primer, a large excess of all four deoxynucleoside triphosphates (deoxyadenosine triphosphate, deoxyguanosine triphosphate, deoxycytidine triphosphate, deoxythymidine triphosphate [dATP, dGTP, dCTP, dTTP]), DNA polymerase, and a small amount of a dideoxynucleotide triphosphate (ddNTP) analogous to one of the four DNA molecules

To enable detection of the DNA fragments, label the primer at the 5′ end or include a labeled deoxynucleotide triphosphate (dNTP) in the reaction mixture

The ddNTP stops transcription when it is incorporated into the growing chain because it has no 3′ OH

Subject the reaction products to gel electrophoresis and autoradiography, and read the sequence from the band patterns (see Fig. 4.3)

**Describe the functionality of polymerase chain reaction (PCR).**

Used to synthesize many copies of a desired fragment of DNA

**Describe the steps in PCR.**

DNA is denatured, or "melted," by heating to generate two separate strands

During cooling, excess primers anneal to a specific sequence on each strand to be amplified

Heat-stable DNA polymerase replicates the DNA sequence following each primer

All the above steps are repeated many times

**PCR can be used to detect what level of genetic mutation?**

Single base pair mutation

**What are the uses of DNA/protein cloning?**

To amplify and obtain a large quantity for study

**What vectors are used to clone DNA?**

Bacteriophage, plasmid

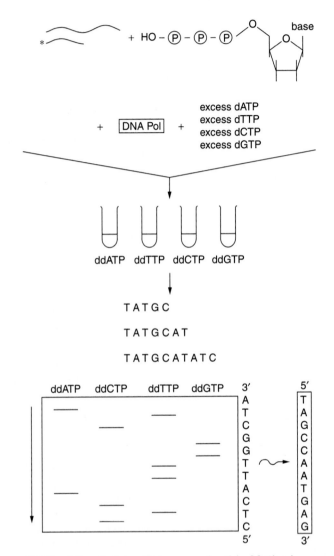

**Figure 4.3**   Sanger Dideoxynucleotide Method.

**Describe the steps involved in cloning DNA and/or protein.**

Cleave the DNA that is to be cloned and the DNA of the vector with the same restriction endonuclease so as to create "sticky ends"

Attach the foreign DNA to the vector by treatment with DNA ligase, thus producing recombinant DNA

Transform bacterial cells by incubating them with the vector containing the recombinant DNA

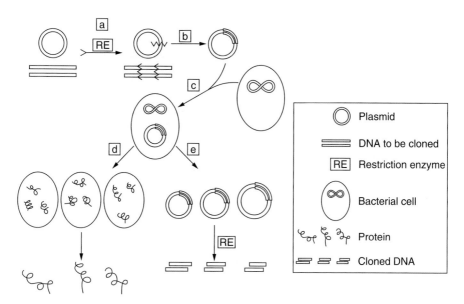

**Figure 4.4** Cloning DNA and Protein. (a) Plasmid and DNA cleaved by the same restriction enzyme; (b) Ligate plasmid DNA and foreign DNA; (c) Transform bacterial cell with plasmid; (d) To obtain protein, grow cultures that allow expression of cloned gene and isolate protein; (e) Isolate plasmids, cleave with restriction endonuclease and isolate cloned DNA.

Plate the transformed bacterial cells to produce individual colonies

Identify and select the colonies containing the recombinant DNA using a probe; isolate and culture those colonies

Isolate and characterize the recombinant DNA, or protein expressed from the recombinant DNA, from the bacterial cells

## CELL CYCLE

| | |
|---|---|
| **What are the phases of the cell cycle?** | $G_1$, S, $G_2$, and M (G = gap, S = synthesis, M = mitosis) |
| **What happens in the $G_1$ phase?** | The cell prepares to initiate DNA synthesis; chromosomes begin to unfold and form euchromatin |

| | |
|---|---|
| The rate of cell division is inversely proportional to the length of what phase of the cell cycle? | $G_1$ |
| Resting or differentiated cells are considered to be in what stage of the cell cycle? | $G_0$ of the $G_1$ phase |
| What roles do the retinoblastoma tumor suppressor protein (pRb) and E2F play in the cell cycle? | E2F is a positive transcription factor that allows the cell to progress into the S phase of the cell cycle. pRb is a protein that if pRb is not phosphorylated, then pRb inactivates E2F by binding to it. When pRb is phosphorylated, pRb releases E2F and the cell is allowed to progress into the S phase of the cell cycle. |
| Mutations in pRb are associated with what types of malignancies? | Retinoblastomas, osteosarcomas |
| What happens in the S phase? | Replication of DNA (DNA doubles in a semiconservative manner) |
| What happens in the $G_2$ phase? | The cell synthesizes the RNA and proteins that are required for mitosis to proceed; chromatin recondenses to form heterochromatin |
| Name the four stages of mitosis. | Prophase, metaphase, anaphase, telophase |
| Methotrexate acts upon which phase of the cell cycle? | S phase |

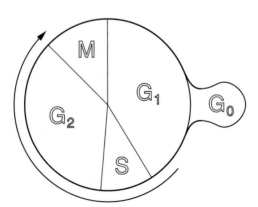

**Figure 4.5**   Cell Cycle.

**Describe methotrexate's mechanism of action.**

It is a folic acid analog, inhibiting dihydrofolate reductase, which results in decreased deoxytrimethyl phosphate (dTMP) along with decreased DNA and protein synthesis.

**What is methotrexate used to treat?**

Rheumatoid arthritis, psoriasis, lymphomas, leukemias, sarcomas, and ectopic pregnancy

**What is a common side effect associated with methotrexate use?**

Myelosuppression

**Is this toxicity reversible?**

Yes, it can be reversed with leucovorin (folinic acid)—termed leucovorin rescue

**5-Flourouracil (5-FU) acts upon which phase of the cell cycle?**

S phase

**What is the mechanism of action of 5-FU?**

It is a pyrimidine analog which is converted to 5F-dUMP. This then combines with folic acid. The combination inhibits thymidylate synthase, which decreases dTMP along with DNA and protein synthesis.

**What is 5-FU used to treat?**

Solid tumors, basal cell carcinomas

**What is a common side effect associated with 5-FU use?**

Myelosuppression ("if you're forced into guessin', say myelosuppression" with the anticancer drugs)

**Is this toxicity reversible?**

No, this is a major difference between methotrexate and 5-FU

**6-Mercaptopurine (6-MP) acts upon which phase of the cell cycle?**

S phase, indirectly

**What is 6-MP's mechanism of action?**

6-MP blocks purine synthesis, thus decreasing DNA synthesis

**What enzyme activates 6-MP?**

Hypoxanthine-guanine phosphoribosyl transferase, HGPRTase (the same enzyme which is deficient in Lesch-Nyhan syndrome)

**What is 6-MP used to treat?**

Leukemia and some lymphomas

**What are some common toxicities associated with 6-MP use?**

Bone marrow, gastrointestinal (GI) system, and liver toxicities

| | |
|---|---|
| Azathioprine is a derivative of what drug? | 6-MP |
| What is the mechanism of action of azathioprine? | Interferes with the synthesis of nucleic acids |
| What is azathioprine used to treat? | It is used as an immunosuppressant for transplantations and autoimmune disorders |
| In what phase of the cell cycle does bleomycin work? | $G_2$ phase |
| Describe bleomycin's mechanism of action. | Intercalates DNA and induces free radicals, which create DNA strand breaks |
| What is bleomycin used to treat? | Lymphomas, testicular cancer |
| What are some toxicities of bleomycin? | Myelosuppression, pulmonary fibrosis |
| In what phase of the cell cycle do the vinca alkaloids (vincristine and vinblastine) work? | M phase |
| What is the mechanism of action of the vinca alkaloids? | Bind to tubulin and block the polymerization of microtubules, thus not allowing the mitotic spindle form |
| What are the vinca alkaloids used to treat? | Lymphoma (vincristine is part of the mechlorethamine, oncovin, procarbazine, prednisone [MOPP] regimen), choriocarcinoma, Wilms' tumor |
| What are the toxicities associated with the use of vinca alkaloids? | Paralytic ileus and neurotoxicity with vincristine, myelosuppression with vinblastine |
| What is the mechanism of action of paclitaxel? | Binds to tubulin and overstabilizes the mitotic spindle, which does not allow the breakdown of the spindle (therefore mitosis gets stuck in metaphase) |
| What is paclitaxel used to treat? | Breast and ovarian cancer |
| What is the main toxicity associated with paclitaxel use? | Myelosuppression |

## DNA AND REPLICATION

**What is semiconservative replication?**

The process by which DNA replicates itself; the two strands are pulled apart and each strand acts as a complement to the newly transcribed DNA (therefore each new DNA is half of the original copy)

**What is an origin of replication?**

The site at which DNA replication begins (in prokaryotes replication begins at a single nucleotide sequence, whereas in eukaryotes replication begins at multiple sites along the DNA helix)

**What is a replication fork?**

A replication fork is where the two strands of DNA are unwinding and separating, creating a "V," which is where active synthesis is taking place

**Is replication of DNA bidirectional or unidirectional?**

Replication of DNA is bidirectional (meaning the replication forks move in both directions away from the origin)

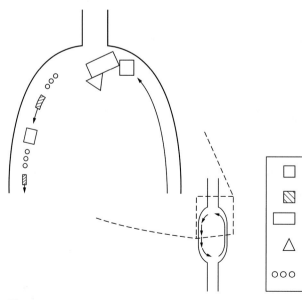

**Figure 4.6** DNA Replication.

**What three prepriming complex proteins are required for the formation of a replication fork?**

DNA protein

Binds to specific nucleotide sequences at the origin of replication, usually where the parental strand is rich in AT base pairs, causing the DNA strands to separate

Single-stranded binding protein

Stabilizes the single-stranded DNA

DNA helicase

Forces the DNA strands apart

**Which enzymes relieve supercoils in DNA?**

Topoisomerases

**Describe the action of DNA topoisomerase I.**

Cuts a single strand of the DNA helix, thus relieving a supercoil

**Describe the function of DNA topoisomerase II.**

Creates breaks in both strands of DNA

**What is the mechanism of action of etoposide?**

Inhibits topoisomerase II and increases DNA degradation

**What is etoposide used to treat?**

Testicular cancer and oat cell carcinoma of the lung (small cell carcinoma)

**What are some toxicities associated with etoposide?**

Myelosuppression, alopecia, GI irritation, and peripheral neurotoxicity

**What is the function of DNA polymerase in replication?**

To copy the DNA templates by catalyzing the step-by-step addition of deoxyribonucleotide units to a DNA chain

**What does DNA polymerase need to synthesize a chain of DNA?**

All four activated precursors (i.e., dATP, dGTP, dTTP, dCTP) and $Mg^{2+}$

Primer chain with a free 3'-OH group

DNA template

**In what direction does DNA polymerase read the parental nucleotide sequence?**

3' to 5' direction (thus DNA replication takes place in the 5' to 3' direction)

**What is the leading strand?**

The strand that is copied in the direction of the advancing replication fork, and is synthesized continuously

| | |
|---|---|
| **What is the lagging strand?** | The strand that is copied in the opposite direction of the advancing replication fork, and is synthesized rather discontinuously (thus creating small fragments of DNA called Okazaki fragments) |
| **What links the Okazaki fragments together to form a continuous strand of DNA?** | DNA ligase |
| **What does DNA polymerase require to begin synthesis of a new strand?** | RNA primer (made by primase in prokaryotes) |
| **Which DNA polymerase is involved in the replication of DNA in prokaryotes?** | DNA polymerase III |
| **Which DNA polymerases are involved in replication of DNA in eukaryotes?** | DNA polymerase $\alpha$ synthesizes RNA primer and replicates lagging strand<br><br>DNA polymerases $\beta$ and $\varepsilon$ are repair polymerases<br><br>DNA polymerase $\delta$ replicates the leading strand<br><br>DNA polymerase $\gamma$ is the mitochondrial polymerase |
| **What is cytarabine's mechanism of action?** | DNA polymerase inhibitor |
| **What is cytarabine used to treat?** | Leukemia, non-Hodgkin's lymphoma |
| **List the common toxicities associated with cytarabine use.** | Thrombocytopenia, leucopenia, and megaloblastic anemia |
| **How are errors in base matching repaired?** | DNA polymerase has a 3' to 5' exonuclease activity (which releases one nucleotide at a time), allowing the detection and removal of mismatched base pairs (hence "editing")—this process is in eukaryotes |
| **What does DNA loop around to condense itself?** | Positively-charged histones (H2A, H2B, H3, H4) |
| **What structure does the aforementioned complex create?** | Nucleosome beads |
| **What protein bridges adjacent nucleosome beads to form 30-nm fiber?** | H1 histones |
| **What is chromatin?** | Condensed DNA looped twice around histone "beads" or DNA plus histones |

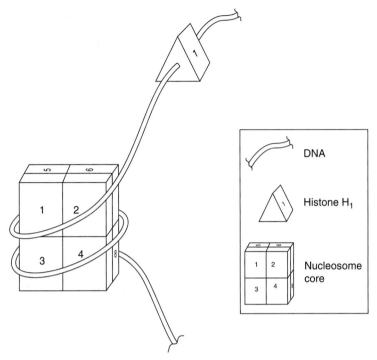

**Figure 4.7** Nucleosome Bead.

**What is heterochromatin?**

The more condensed, transcriptionally inactive form of chromatin

**What is euchromatin?**

The less condensed, transcriptionally active form of chromatin (remember "eu" means "true," so euchromatin is "truly" transcribed)

**What are some of the ways in which DNA can become damaged?**

Ultraviolet light exposure, extremes of pH, increased temperature, and alkylating agents

**Name four DNA repair defect syndromes.**

Xeroderma pigmentosum (exposure to UV light), ataxia-telangiectasia (exposure to x-rays), Bloom's syndrome (exposure to radiation), and Fanconi anemia (exposure to intercalating agents)

**What is a transition mutation?**

When a purine is substituted for a purine or a pyrimidine is substituted for a pyrimidine

| | |
|---|---|
| **What is a transversion mutation?** | When a purine is substituted for a pyrimidine or vice versa (think transconversion) |
| **Name some features of the genetic code.** | It is unambiguous (each codon specifies only one amino acid), degenerate (more than one codon codes for a single amino acid), comma-less and nonoverlapping, and universal |
| **What is a silent DNA mutation?** | A mutation in a codon that results in a new codon which codes for the same amino acid (often the third base in the codon is changed, i.e., the wobble position) |
| **What is a missense DNA mutation?** | A mutation in a codon that results in a new codon which codes for a different amino acid |
| **What is a nonsense DNA mutation?** | A mutation that creates a stop codon, and prematurely terminates the translation of a coded protein |
| **What is a frameshift DNA mutation?** | A mutation that inserts or deletes bases resulting in a misreading of the genetic code downstream of the mutation; usually resulting in a premature stop codon |
| **What is the order of severity of the aforementioned DNA mutations?** | Nonsense/frameshift mutation > missense mutation > silent mutation |

## RNA AND TRANSCRIPTION

| | |
|---|---|
| **What is transcription?** | The conversion of DNA to RNA (transcripts of certain regions of DNA) |
| **What are the three major types of RNA?** | Ribosomal RNA (rRNA), messenger RNA (mRNA), transfer RNA (tRNA) |
| **Name the different types of eukaryotic RNA polymerases.** | RNA polymerase I makes rRNA, RNA polymerase II makes mRNA, and RNA polymerase III makes tRNA (remember R-M-T: rRNA is rampant, mRNA is massive, tRNA is tiny. I, II, and III are numbered as their products are used in protein synthesis) |

**What are the different types of prokaryotic RNA polymerases?**

One RNA polymerase makes all prokaryotic RNA

**What are the three phases of transcription?**

Initiation, elongation, and termination (initiation begins with RNA polymerase II binding to a specific region of DNA known as the promoter region—usually a stretch of about six nucleotides known as the TATA box [TATAAT], about 8–10 nucleotides upstream from the start of transcription)

**In what direction does transcription take place?**

$5'$ to $3'$

**Describe the elongation phase.**

The DNA is unwound with negative supercoils relieved by gyrases and topoisomerase II (both of these cut two strands of DNA) and positive supercoils relieved by topoisomerase I (this cuts only one strand of DNA)

**What pyrophosphates are required for DNA elongation to occur?**

dATP, dTTP, dCTP, dGTP

**How does RNA polymerase differ from DNA polymerase?**

RNA polymerase does not require a primer and has no exonuclease or endonuclease activity (no proofreading)

**Describe the termination phase.**

A termination signal is reached which ends transcription

**What are some antibiotics that prevent cell growth by inhibiting RNA synthesis?**

Rifampin (DNA-dependent RNA polymerase inhibitor), dactinomycin (acts by binding to the DNA template and interfering with the movement of RNA polymerase along the DNA)

**Describe the eukaryotic promoter regions.**

A TATA box, which is near the site of transcription, and a CAAT box, which is more distant

**What are enhancers?**

DNA sequences that increase the rate of transcription initiation by RNA polymerase II by binding transcription factors

**Are enhancers position-dependent or position-independent?**

Position-independent (meaning that they can be located upstream, within, or downstream of the area being transcribed)

| | |
|---|---|
| What is $\alpha$-amanitine's mechanism of action? | Forms a tight complex with the RNA polymerase II, thus inhibiting mRNA synthesis and eventually protein synthesis ($\alpha$-amanitine is a poison produced by the *Amanita phalloides* mushroom) |
| What modifies the primary (original) transcript of tRNA and rRNA? | Ribonuclease |
| Is prokaryotic or eukaryotic mRNA posttranscriptionally modified? | Only eukaryotic mRNA; prokaryotic mRNA is identical to its primary transcript, heterogeneous nuclear RNA (hnRNA) |
| Where in the cell is mRNA transcribed? | Nucleus of eukaryotes, cytosol of prokaryotes |
| Where in the cell is mRNA translated? | Cytosol |
| What three modifications does mRNA undergo? | Capping of the 5' end, addition of a poly-A tail to the 3' end, and removal of introns |
| What is an intron? | Intervening sequences that do not code for proteins |
| What is an exon? | Sequences that code for proteins; they are spliced together to form mature mRNA |
| What do small nuclear RNAs (snRNAs) do? | They are part of small nuclear ribonucleoproteins (snRNPs), which facilitate the splicing of exon segments |
| How is systemic lupus erythematous (SLE) associated with snRNPs? | SLE results from an autoimmune response in which the patient produces antibodies against snRNPs (this is one of the associations of SLE, not the definitive association) |

## TRANSLATION

| | |
|---|---|
| What is the dogma of expression for genetic information? | DNA to RNA to protein (the first step being transcription, the second step being translation) |
| In what direction does DNA replication, transcription, and translation occur? | 5' to 3' |
| What is a codon? | Three nucleotides (bases) set in a particular order that correspond to a protein |

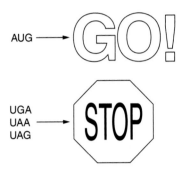

AUG

UGA
UAA
UAG

**Figure 4.8**   The Codons.

What is the usual start codon
in prokaryotes?

AUG—this codes for a methionine,
which is usually formulated

Name the stop codons.

UGA, UAA, UAG (remember U Go
Away, U Are Away, and U Are
Gone)—these codons signify to the
protein to stop translating the
protein

What reads the mRNA codon and
delivers the correct amino acid?

tRNA

Describe the shape of tRNA.

Cloverleaf, with an anticodon area to
read the mRNA's codon

Where on the tRNA is the attachment
for each specific amino acid?

The 3′ end

What does aminoacyl-tRNA synthetase do?

Catalyzes a two-step reaction that
results in the covalent attachment of
an amino acid to the 3′ end of the
corresponding tRNA (this enzyme
requires ATP); basically it recognizes
the correct tRNA to the
corresponding amino acid

Describe the structure of ribosomes
in prokaryotes and eukaryotes.

Prokaryotic ribosomes have two
subunits, one being the 50S subunit
and the other, the 30S subunit;
eukaryotic ribosomes have
two subunits also, one being the
60S subunit and the other, the 40S
subunit.

What are the binding sites on the
ribosome for the tRNA molecule called?

The A and P sites

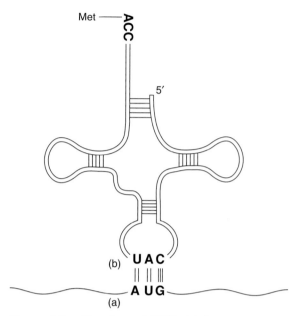

**Figure 4.9**  Structure of tRNA. (a) Codon; (b) Anticodon.

| | |
|---|---|
| **Explain how the A and P sites work.** | They cover two neighboring codons; the A site binds an incoming aminoacyl tRNA and the P site binds the next aminoacyl tRNA to be added |
| **In what direction are proteins constructed?** | N terminus to C terminus |
| **Where in the cell are ribosomes located?** | In eukaryotes, there are free ribosomes in the cytosol (responsible for making proteins that will stay within the cell) and rough ribosomes located in the endoplasmic reticulum (responsible for making proteins that will be secreted extracellularly, incorporated into the plasma membrane, or included within lysosomes) |
| **How many high-energy phosphate bonds are needed to add one amino acid to a growing peptide chain?** | Four bonds (two ATP for the aminoacyl-tRNA synthetase reaction + one GTP for binding the aminoacyl tRNA to the A site + one GTP for the translocation step) |

| | |
|---|---|
| Describe the "wobble" theory. | The hypothesis that if the first two nucleotides in a codon are similar and the third nucleotide is different; often the same amino acid will be coded |
| What is meant by polycistronic mRNA? | When a single mRNA has many coding regions, each with its own initiation site |
| What is meant by monocistronic mRNA? | When an mRNA codes for only one specific polypeptide |
| Is prokaryotic mRNA polycistronic or monocistronic? | Polycistronic (remember prokaryotes, polycistronic) |
| Is eukaryotic mRNA polycistronic or monocistronic? | Monocistronic |
| What are the three stages of translation? | Initiation, elongation, and termination |
| What is the enzyme that catalyzes the formation of peptide bonds? | Peptidyl transferase |
| What is a polysome? | A complex consisting of one mRNA and multiple ribosomes translating the message |
| How are proteins modified following translation? | Proteins may be phosphorylated, glycosylated, acylated, hydroxylated, have disulfide bonds added, and undergo enzymatic cleavage |
| List some common antibiotics that act on the bacterial 30S ribosomal subunit. | Aminoglycosides (i.e., streptomycin, gentamicin, tobramycin, amikacin) are bactericidal and tetracyclines (i.e., tetracycline, doxycycline, demeclocycline, minocycline) are bacteriostatic |
| List some common antibiotics that act on the bacterial 50S subunit. | Chloramphenicol, erythromycin/ macrolides, lincomycin, clindamycin, streptogramins (i.e., quinupristin, dalfopristin), and linezolid |
| What is the mechanism of action for chloramphenicol? | It inhibits the bacterial 50S peptidyl transferase—chloramphenicol is bacteriostatic |
| What is the mechanism of action for erythromycin/macrolides? | They inhibit protein synthesis by blocking translocation via their binding to the 23S rRNA of the 50S ribosomal subunit—these antibiotics are bacteriostatic |

| | |
|---|---|
| What is the mechanism of action for clindamycin? | It blocks peptide bond formation at the bacterial 50S ribosomal subunit—clindamycin is bacteriostatic |

## CANCER DRUGS

| | |
|---|---|
| What is the mechanism by which busulfan works? | Alkylating DNA, resulting in its deactivation |
| What is busulfan used to treat? | Chronic myelogenous leukemia (CML) |
| What are the major side effects associated with busulfan use? | Hyperpigmentation, pulmonary fibrosis |
| Describe the mechanism by which cyclophosphamide works. | Following hepatic bioactivation, it is an alkylating agent that cross-links DNA at guanine N-7 |
| What is cyclophosphamide used to treat? | Breast cancer, non-Hodgkin's lymphoma |
| What are cyclophosphamide's toxicities? | Myelosuppression, hemorrhagic cystitis (preventable with the use of mesna, which reacts with the urotoxic metabolites) |
| What is the mechanism by which the nitrosoureas (i.e., carmustine, lomustine, streptozocin) work? | Alkylating DNA |
| What are nitrosoureas used to treat? | Brain tumors (because they can cross the blood-brain barrier) |
| What is a common toxicity associated with the use of nitrosoureas? | Central nervous system (CNS), they can cause ataxia and/or dizziness |
| What is the mechanism by which cisplatin works? | Alkylating DNA |
| What is cisplatin used to treat? | Bladder, ovary, testicular, and lung small cell cancer |
| What are the common toxicities of cisplatin? | Renal toxicity and acoustic nerve damage |
| What is the mechanism of doxorubicin's action? | Intercalating DNA, thus creating a break and causing a decrease in replication while generating toxic radicals |

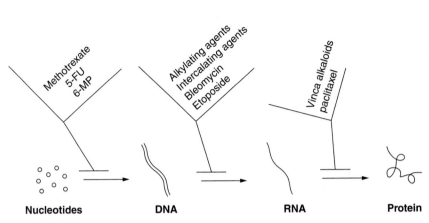

**Figure 4.10**   Cancer Drugs.

| | |
|---|---|
| **What is doxorubicin used to treat?** | Hodgkin's lymphoma, sarcomas, and solid tumors (lung, ovary, breast, colon) |
| **What are some toxicities of doxorubicin?** | Cardiotoxicity, myelosuppression, alopecia |

# CHAPTER 5

# Genetics

## OVERVIEW

| | |
|---|---|
| In autosomal dominant (AD) inheritance, are males or females more affected? | Both are equally affected |
| What genes are usually affected in disorders with AD inheritance? | Structural genes |
| What occurs in an amorphic gene mutation? | Gene fails to work |
| What occurs in a hypomorphic gene mutation? | Gene works poorly |
| What occurs in a neomorphic gene mutation? | Gene functions in an inappropriate manner |
| What occurs in a hypermorphic gene mutation? | Gene functions in excess of its normal function |
| What occurs in an antimorphic gene mutation? | Gene is mutated and affects various systems in the body |

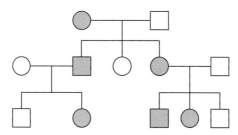

**Figure 5.1**  Autosomal Dominant Pedigree.

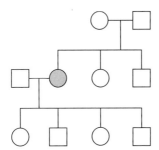

**Figure 5.2** Autosomal Recessive Pedigree.

| | |
|---|---|
| **Name some common AD disorders.** | Huntington's disease, familial hypercholesterolemia type IIa, neurofibromatosis I and II, tuberous sclerosis, adult polycystic kidney disease (APKD), Marfan's syndrome, hereditary spherocytosis, familial adenomatous polyposis (FAP), von Hippel-Lindau syndrome, von Willebrand's disease, all multiple endocrine neoplasia (MEN) syndromes, achondroplasia, familial hypocalciuric hypercalcemia |
| **Two carriers of a lethal autosomal recessive (AR) disorder have a child. What is the probability that the child will die as a result of this disorder?** | 25% |
| **What is the probability that their child will be healthy but also a carrier?** | 66% |
| **What is meant by the term horizontal transmission?** | A disease phenotype is seen in multiple siblings, usually with no earlier generations affected |
| **What is consanguinity?** | The mating of related individuals, which may be suspected when analyzing the cause of rare AR disorders |
| **Name some characteristics of AR traits/disorders.** | Often due to enzyme deficiencies, often more severe than AD disorders, and patients often present in childhood |
| **Are males or females more commonly affected in AR disorders?** | Males and females are equally affected |
| **Are males or females more commonly affected in X-linked recessive disorders?** | Males (remember, males only have one X-chromosome) |

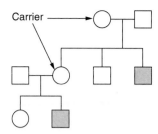

**Figure 5.3**   X-Linked Recessive Pedigree.

| | |
|---|---|
| **What is lyonization?** | The normal phenomenon that wherever there are two or more haploid sets of X-linked genes in each cell, all but one of the genes are randomly inactivated and have no phenotypic expression |
| **What is the importance of lyonization in X-linked disorders?** | It explains the more variable expression of X-linked traits in women than in men |
| **Name some common X-linked recessive disorders.** | Fragile X, hemophilia A and B, Duchenne's muscular dystrophy, Fabry's, glucose-6-phosphate dehydrogenase deficiency, Hunter's syndrome, Lesch-Nyhan syndrome, Bruton's agammaglobulinemia, Wiskott-Aldrich syndrome |
| **What is the main feature of mitochondrial inheritance?** | Transmission of the disorder is only through the mother |
| **What does variable expression mean?** | The nature and severity of the phenotype varies from one individual to another |
| **What does incomplete penetrance mean?** | Not all individuals with a mutant genotype will show the mutant phenotype |

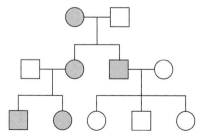

**Figure 5.4**   Mitochondrial Inheritance Pedigree.

**What is pleiotropy?** The ability of a single allele to have more than one distinguishable effect

**What is imprinting?** Differences in a phenotype depending on whether a mutation occurs in the mother's or father's alleles

**Give two examples of imprinting.** Angelman's syndrome (deletion in the maternal allele of chromosome 15q12), Prader-Willi syndrome (deletion in the paternal allele of chromosome 15q12)

**Name the clinical manifestations of Angelman's syndrome.** Mental retardation, ataxia, seizures, strange affect, inappropriate laughter (hence, the happy puppet syndrome)

**Name the clinical manifestations of Prader-Willi syndrome.** Hypotonia, poor infant feeding followed by childhood obesity, hyperphagia, delayed psychomotor development

**What is anticipation?** The severity of a disorder worsens or the disorder manifests earlier in future generations

**What is an example of a disease that exhibits anticipation?** Huntington's disease

**Where is the mutation in Huntington's disease?** Chromosome 4p (remember "Hunting 4 food")

**Name some features of Huntington's disease.** Autosomal dominant disorder showcasing anticipation, usually presenting in the ages of 20–50 years, and affected patients can develop depression, chorea, jerky hyperkinetic movements, caudate atrophy (disease progression is directly proportional to the size of the lateral ventricles)

**What is loss of heterozygosity?** If an individual has a mutation or develops a mutation in a tumor suppressor gene, then the other allele must be deleted or mutated before a neoplasm can develop

**Do oncogenes show loss of heterozygosity?** No

**Name some characteristics of X-linked dominant inheritance.** Can be transmitted through either parent, all female offspring of an affected father will also be affected, males are generally more severely affected than females

| | |
|---|---|
| **Name some X-linked dominant disorders.** | Xg blood group, vitamin D-resistant (hypophosphatemic) rickets, Rett syndrome, pseudohypoparathyroidism, ornithine transcarbamylase deficiency |
| **What is a dominant negative mutation?** | The dominant allele, even in a heterozygote state, produces a nonfunctional protein that exerts its effect on the normal allele and does not allow the production of a functional protein (hence, its dominance over the functional allele) |
| **What is linkage disequilibrium?** | The tendency for certain alleles at two different loci on the chromosome to occur together more often than by chance |
| **What is mosaicism?** | When different cells in the body express different alleles (i.e., X-linked inactivation in which a certain subset of cells inactivates one X-chromosome and another subset of cells inactivate the other X-chromosome) |
| **What is gene flow?** | Exchange of genes among different populations |
| **When is a concordance study of twins used?** | To determine heritability of multifactorial traits |
| **What is the equation used to determine this heritability?** | Heritability $= C_{mz} - C_{dz}/1 - C_{dz}$ $C_{mz}$ is the concordance in monozygotic twins $C_{dz}$ is the concordance in dizygotic twins |
| **What is the Hardy-Weinberg equation?** | $p^2 + 2pq + q^2 = 1$     $p + q = 1$ p and q are separate alleles; 2pq = heterozygote prevalence |
| **What is the Hardy-Weinberg equation used to calculate in recessive disease models?** | Carrier frequency |
| **What are the four assumptions of Hardy-Weinberg population genetics?** | No mutations Random mating No migration No selection |
| **What can cause allele frequency to increase in a population?** | Heterozygote advantage, genetic bottleneck, migration, new mutation |

# CHROMOSOMAL ABNORMALITIES

| | |
|---|---|
| What is aneuploidy? | The state of having an abnormal number of chromosomes, not an exact multiple of the haploid number |
| What is polyploidy? | The state of having three or more haploid sets of chromosomes |
| What is the most common cause of polyploidy? | Polyspermy or egg fertilization by two sperms, accounts for two-thirds of the cases |
| What is a reciprocal translocation? | The mutual exchange of chromosomal material between two different chromosomes |
| Will an individual with a balanced reciprocal translocation be phenotypically normal? | Yes (but their offspring is at increased risk of having an unbalanced translocation) |
| What is a Robertsonian translocation? | A translocation in which the centromeres of two acrocentric chromosomes appear to have fused, forming an abnormal chromosome consisting of the long arms of two different chromosomes |
| What is the difference between a terminal deletion and interstitial deletion? | A terminal deletion involves the end of a chromosome but an interstitial deletion involves a region within a chromosome. |
| What type of genetic mutation may result in trisomy of a particular chromosomal segment? | Duplication |
| What is the difference between a pericentric inversion and paracentric inversion? | A pericentric inversion includes the centromere and a paracentric inversion does not include the centromere. |
| What is a ring chromosome? | A chromosome with ends joined to form a circular structure; the ring form is abnormal in humans but the normal form of the chromosome in certain bacteria. |
| What percentage of live births have a chromosomal abnormality? | 0.5% |
| What percentage of clinically recognized pregnancies result in spontaneous abortion? | 15% |

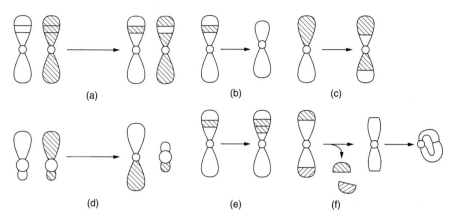

**Figure 5.5** Chromosomal Structural Abnormalities. (a) Reciprocal Translocation; (b) Deletion; (c) Duplication; (d) Robertsonian Translocation; (e) Inversion; (f) Ring Conversion.

| | |
|---|---|
| Chromosomal abnormalities are implicated in what percentage of spontaneous first-trimester abortions? | 50% |
| What disorder is characterized by congenital mental retardation, flat facial profile, duodenal atresia, and congenital heart disease? | Down syndrome (trisomy 21) |
| This disorder is associated with what maternal parameter? | Advanced maternal age |
| What is the most common cause of this disorder? | Meiotic nondisjunction of homologous chromosomes |
| What percentage of cases are a result of unbalanced Robertsonian translocations? | 3% |
| What is the incidence of this disorder? | 1:800 |
| What disorder is characterized by severe mental retardation, clenched fists with overlapping digits, and rocker-bottom feet? | Edwards' syndrome (trisomy 18) |
| What is the prognosis of an individual with this disorder? | Incompatible with life beyond 2 years of age |
| What is the incidence of this disorder? | 1:8000 |
| What disorder is characterized by severe mental retardation, microcephaly with microphthalmia, cleft palate/cleft lip, and polydactyly? | Patau's syndrome (trisomy 13) |
| What is the prognosis of an individual with this disorder? | Death commonly by 1 year of age |

| | |
|---|---|
| What is the incidence of this disorder? | 1:6000 |
| Describe the symptoms of Klinefelter's syndrome. | XXY male with testicular atrophy, gynecomastia, eunuchoid body shape, and female hair distribution |
| What is the cause of Klinefelter's syndrome? | Meiotic nondisjunction of the sex chromosomes |
| What is the gonadal state of individuals with this disorder? | Hypogonadism (but at increased risk of developing breast cancer) |
| What is the incidence of this disorder? | 1:850 |
| What are the symptoms of Turner's syndrome? | XO female with short stature, ovarian dysgenesis, webbing of the neck, and primary amenorrhea |
| Individuals with Turner's syndrome are at increased risk to have what cardiac abnormality? | Coarctation of the aorta |
| What is the incidence of Turner's syndrome? | 1:3000 |
| What are the symptoms of an individual with double Y? | XYY males who are phenotypically normal, but usually tall with severe acne |
| What is the incidence of this disorder? | 1:1000 (increased frequency among inmates of penal institutions) |

## GENETIC DISORDERS

| | |
|---|---|
| What disorder characterized by macro-orchidism, a long face with large jaw, large everted ears, and autism is the second most common cause of congenital mental retardation? | Fragile X syndrome |
| What genetic abnormality is associated with this disorder? | Progressive expansion of an unstable DNA triple repeat on the X-chromosome |
| One would like to run an electrophoresis gel to separate the abnormal X-chromosome from the normal X-chromosome in a carrier female. Relative to the normal X-chromosome, would the abnormal X-chromosome run a longer or shorter distance on the gel? | Shorter distance because the expanded abnormal X-chromosome would be molecularly larger than the normal X-chromosome |

| | |
|---|---|
| **What method is normally used in diagnosis?** | Lymphocyte culturing in either folate-deficient medium or with chemical agents such as methotrexate; histological analysis revealing >4% of metaphase chromosomes with a characteristic break is diagnostic |
| **Describe the inheritance pattern of this disorder.** | X-linked recessive |
| **What is the incidence of this disorder?** | 1:1500 males |
| **What disorder is characterized by severe mental retardation, microcephaly, cardiac abnormalities, and laryngeal malformation?** | Cri du chat syndrome (i.e., cry of the cat) |
| **Describe the genetic abnormality associated with this disorder.** | Congenial deletion of the short arm of chromosome 5 (46, XX or XY, 5p-) |
| **What are the symptoms of von Recklinghausen's disease (NFT1)?** | Café-au-lait spots, neural tumors, Lisch nodules, and increased tumor susceptibility |
| **This disorder is associated with a mutation on which chromosome?** | Long arm of chromosome 17 (remember there are 17 letters in von Recklinghausen) |
| **Describe the inheritance pattern of von Recklinghausen's disease.** | Autosomal dominant |
| **What is the incidence of von Recklinghausen's disease?** | 1:3000 |
| **What disease is characterized by cystic bilateral enlargement of the kidneys, hematuria, hypertension, and progressive renal failure?** | APKD |
| **This disorder is associated with a mutation on what chromosome?** | APKD1 gene on chromosome 16 |
| **What is the inheritance pattern of this disorder?** | Autosomal dominant |
| **What is the inheritance pattern of the juvenile form of this disorder?** | Autosomal recessive |
| **Marfan's syndrome is caused by a mutation in the gene encoding for what protein?** | Fibrillin (FBN), a component of connective tissue |
| **The abnormality in Marfan's syndrome is an example of what type of gene mutation?** | Antimorphic gene mutation |
| **Where is this gene located?** | FBN-1 is located on chromosome 15 |

| | |
|---|---|
| What are the clinical manifestations of Marfan's syndrome? | Tall stature, long and thin fingers, scoliosis, subluxation of the lenses, and cystic medial necrosis of the aorta (leading to aortic incompetence and dissecting aortic aneurysms) |
| How is Marfan's syndrome inherited? | Autosomal dominant pattern |
| What are the symptoms of Velo-Cardio-Facial syndrome? | Cleft palate, mental retardation, hypernasal speech, and cardiac abnormalities |
| What type of genetic mutation is associated with Velo-Cardio-Facial syndrome? | Microdeletion on chromosome 22q |
| What is the incidence of Velo-Cardio-Facial syndrome? | 1:3000 |

## CANCER GENETICS

| | |
|---|---|
| Describe the multistage model for carcinogenesis. | Cancer is not a single event; rather, it is a multistage process in which an initial mutation in a somatic cell is followed by subsequent mutations and alterations which accumulate over time and lead to cancer |
| What is a tumor suppressor gene? | A gene whose function is to suppress cellular proliferation |
| What is the role of a tumor suppressor gene in neoplastic transformation? | It suppresses neoplastic transformation; loss of a tumor suppressor gene (both alleles) through chromosomal aberration leads to heightened susceptibility to neoplastic changes |
| Describe the Knudsen hypothesis. | An explanation for the bilateral (and earlier) occurrence of hereditary retinoblastoma; if one tumor suppressor gene is mutated by inheritance, only one somatic mutation is needed to inactivate the other allele |
| What tumor suppressor gene is implicated in the development of most human cancers? | p53 |
| Where is this tumor suppressor gene located? | 17p |

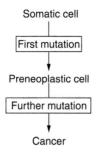

Somatic cell

First mutation

Preneoplastic cell

Further mutation

Cancer

**Figure 5.6**   Knudsen Hypothesis.

| | |
|---|---|
| **What protein does it encode?** | A nucleophosphoprotein that binds DNA and negatively regulates cell division; when it is nonfunctional, cells with damaged DNA are allowed to progress through the cell cycle, possibly accumulating more damage, and predisposing these cells to neoplastic changes |
| **What disorder is a result of germ-line mutations in this tumor suppressor gene?** | Li-Fraumeni syndrome |
| **What cancers occur most commonly in individuals with this disorder?** | Breast cancer, brain tumors, acute leukemia, soft tissue sarcomas, osteosarcoma, and adrenal cortical carcinoma |
| **What disorder is characterized by hemangioblastomas of the retina, cerebellum, and medulla?** | Von Hippel-Lindau disease |
| **This disorder is associated with the deletion of what gene?** | Von Hippel-Lindau tumor suppressor gene |
| **Where is this gene located?** | Chromosome 3p |
| **What disorders are associated with a deletion in the adenomatous polyposis coli (APC) tumor suppressor gene?** | Familial adenomatous polyposis (FAP), Gardner's syndrome, some Turcot's syndrome families, attenuated adenomatous polyposis coli (AAPC) |
| **Where is the APC gene located?** | Chromosome 5q |
| **Describe the function of the APC gene.** | Promotes apoptosis by sequestering the growth stimulatory effects of $\beta$-catenin |
| **The BRCA1 and BRCA2 tumor suppressor genes are implicated in the development of what tumors?** | Breast cancer, ovarian cancer |

| | |
|---|---|
| **Where are these genes located?** | BRCA1 on chromosome 17q, BRCA2 on chromosome 13q |
| **These genes encode for what type of proteins?** | DNA repair regulators |
| **What is the lifetime risk of developing breast cancer for a female with a germ-line mutation of BRCA1?** | 80% |
| **What is the lifetime risk of developing ovarian cancer for a female with a germ-line mutation of BRCA1?** | 60% |
| **What is the lifetime risk of developing breast or ovarian cancer for a female with a germ-line mutation of BRCA1?** | Almost 100% |
| **Does a female with an individual germ-line mutation of BRCA1 or BRCA2 have a greater lifetime risk of developing ovarian cancer?** | BRCA2 |
| **What is an oncogene?** | A gene that codes for a protein involved in cell growth or regulation but may foster malignant processes if mutated or activated by contact with retroviruses |
| **List the proteins that an oncogene may code for.** | Protein kinases, guanosine 5′-triphosphatases (GTPases), nuclear proteins, growth factors |
| **What is the Philadelphia chromosome?** | An abnormal minute chromosome formed by a rearrangement of chromosomes 9 and 22; forms a bcr-abl fusion gene which translates for a protein with abnormal tyrosine kinase activity |
| **The Philadelphia chromosome is found in cultured leukocytes of individuals with what disorder?** | Chronic myelogenous leukemia (CML) |
| **What drug is used to treat this disorder?** | Gleevec |
| **Describe Gleevec's mechanism of action.** | Gleevec is a protein-tyrosine kinase inhibitor that inhibits the bcr-abl tyrosine kinase created by the Philadelphia chromosome; thus, it inhibits proliferation and induces apoptosis in bcr-abl-positive cell line. |

| | |
|---|---|
| **What translocation is associated with Burkitt's lymphoma?** | t(8;14) |
| **What gene is overactivated following this translocation?** | c-myc, a transcription factor essential for mitosis of mammalian cells |
| **What virus may be implicated in the development of Burkitt's lymphoma?** | Epstein-Barr virus |
| **What translocation is associated with follicular lymphoma?** | t(14;18) |
| **What gene is overactivated following this translocation?** | bcl-2, an inhibitor of apoptosis |
| **What translocation is associated with acute myelogenous leukemia (AML) (M3 type)?** | t(15;17) |
| **AML is responsive to treatment with what drug?** | All-trans retinoic acid |
| **What translocation is associated with Ewing's sarcoma?** | t(11;22) (remember, Patrick Ewing wore number 11 + 22 = 33) |
| **What gene is overactivated following this translocation?** | c-myc, a transcription factor essential for mitosis of mammalian cells |
| **What translocation is associated with mantle cell lymphoma?** | t(11;14) |
| **What gene is overactivated following this translocation?** | bcl-1, a promoter of cell cycle progression |
| **What is a carcinogen?** | Any cancer-producing substance |
| **What is the proposed mechanism of action for most carcinogens?** | Cause damage to DNA, and so generate mutations |
| **What test identifies the mutagenicity of a potential carcinogen?** | Ames test |
| **Describe this test.** | A screening test for possible carcinogens using strains of *Salmonella typhimurium* that are unable to synthesize histidine; if the test substance produces mutations that regain the ability to synthesize histidine, the substance is carcinogenic |
| **List the classes of carcinogens.** | Chemical carcinogens, viruses, radiation |

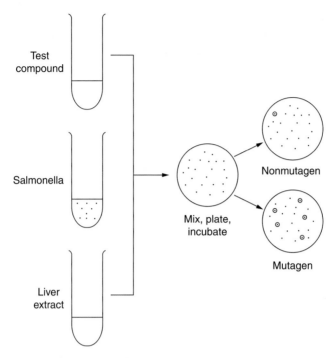

**Figure 5.7**   The Ames Test.

**List the associated carcinogens for the following organs:**

| | |
|---|---|
| Liver | Aflatoxins, vinyl chloride, oral contraceptive pills, Hepatitis B and C viruses, carbon tetrachloride |
| Esophagus | Nitrosamines, tobacco, gastroesophageal reflux disease (GERD) |
| Stomach | Nitrosamines |
| Lung | Tobacco, asbestos |
| Skin | Arsenic, radiation, human herpesvirus-8 (HHV-8) (Kaposi's sarcoma) |
| Bladder | Naphthalene (aniline) dyes, *Schistosoma haematobium* |
| Cervix/penis/anus | Human papilloma virus |
| Blood | Human T-cell lymphotrophic virus type I |

# CHAPTER 6

# Cell Biology and Physiology

## PLASMA MEMBRANE

List the biological ions important to cell physiology.

Sodium, potassium, magnesium, calcium, hydrogen, chloride

What feature of a cell allows for the compartmentalization of biological functions?

Lipid membranes

What substances are the typical constituents of a plasma membrane?

Cholesterol, phospholipids, sphingolipids, glycolipids, proteins

The plasma membrane has what basic molecular structure?

Phospholipid bilayer

Name two important characteristics of a phospholipid.

Polar head, hydrophobic tail

In what organelle are phospholipids synthesized?

Endoplasmic reticulum

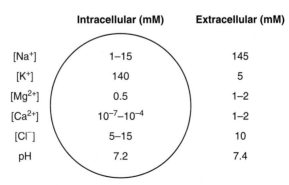

|  | Intracellular (mM) | Extracellular (mM) |
|---|---|---|
| $[Na^+]$ | 1–15 | 145 |
| $[K^+]$ | 140 | 5 |
| $[Mg^{2+}]$ | 0.5 | 1–2 |
| $[Ca^{2+}]$ | $10^{-7}-10^{-4}$ | 1–2 |
| $[Cl^-]$ | 5–15 | 10 |
| pH | 7.2 | 7.4 |

**Figure 6.1** Concentrations of Ions.

| | |
|---|---|
| **What structure(s) do phospholipids spontaneously form when placed in water?** | Micelles or bilayers |
| **The aforementioned structure is formed as a result of what property of water?** | Polarity of water; hydrocarbons, such as phospholipids, placed in water disrupt the ability of water molecules to form hydrogen bonds but bilayer formation allows water to reform these hydrogen bonds |
| **Sphingolipids are an important constituent of what type of tissue?** | Nerve tissue (see the lysosomal storage diseases section) |
| **What chemical force drives the formation of a lipid membrane?** | Hydrophobic interactions between the phospholipid tails; hydrophilic interactions between phospholipids heads and extracellular/cytosolic fluid |
| **What are the four major phospholipids present in the plasma membrane?** | Phosphatidylserine, phosphatidylinositol, phosphatidylcholine, and phosphatidylethanolamine |
| **What two types of lipids are more predominate on the outer leaflet of the bilayer?** | Phosphatidylcholine (lecithin) and sphingomyelin |
| **What two types of lipids are more predominate on the inner leaflet of the bilayer?** | Phosphatidylserine and phosphatidylethanolamine |
| **The sugar component of glycoproteins and glycolipids are usually found on which side of the plasma membrane?** | Extracellular side |
| **The sugar constituent of a glycoprotein is found on which side of the plasma membrane?** | Extracellular side |
| **List the molecules and structures in which lecithin is a component.** | Surfactant (i.e., dipalmitoyl phosphatidylcholine), myelin, red blood cell (RBC) membranes, bile |
| **Deficiency of surfactant is associated with what potentially fatal neonatal disorder?** | Neonatal respiratory distress syndrome (hyaline membrane disease) |
| **What is the treatment of choice for the aforementioned disorder?** | Maternal prenatal administration of betamethasone or artificial surfactant for the infant |
| **What are the two factors that influence the fluidity of the plasma membrane?** | Cholesterol content and the length of the unsaturated fatty chains of the phospholipids |
| **Fluidity of the plasma membrane is crucial to what cellular processes?** | Exocytosis, endocytosis, membrane trafficking, membrane biogenesis |

| | |
|---|---|
| **What groups of molecules can freely diffuse across a lipid membrane?** | Hydrophobic molecules (i.e., $O_2$, $CO_2$, $N_2$, benzene) and small uncharged polar molecules (i.e., $H_2O$, urea, glycerol) |
| **Describe what happens to a cell placed in the following solutions:** | |
| **Hypertonic solution?** | Decreases in size |
| **Isotonic solution?** | No change in size |
| **Hypotonic solution?** | Increases in size |
| **The influx or efflux of molecules across a lipid membrane is dependent on what two factors?** | Permeability of the lipid membrane and driving force |
| **The driving force is directly proportional to what factors?** | For uncharged molecules, driving force is directly proportional to the concentration gradient across the lipid membrane. For charged molecules, the driving force is directly proportional to the concentration gradient and electrochemical gradient across the lipid membrane. |

## MEMBRANE PROTEINS

| | |
|---|---|
| **Name the three classes of membrane proteins.** | Integral proteins (including transmembrane proteins), surface membrane proteins, and inner membrane proteins |

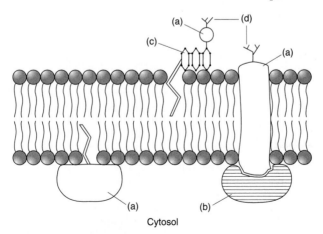

**Figure 6.2** Membrane Proteins. (a) Integral Proteins; (b) Peripheral Proteins; (c) Oligosaccharide; (d) Carbohydrate.

| | |
|---|---|
| Which membrane proteins stabilize the plasma membrane and maintain RBC shape? | Integrins (i.e., spectrin, actin, band 4.1 protein, ankyrin) |
| What disease results from defects in spectrin? | Hereditary spherocytosis |
| Transport proteins belong to which class? | Integral proteins |
| What is the difference between homo-oligomeric and hetero-oligomeric transport proteins? | Homo-oligomeric transport proteins are made up of several copies of the same integral membrane protein whereas hetero-oligomeric transport proteins are made up of several different integral membrane proteins. |
| What role may surface membrane or inner membrane proteins play in transport? | They can associate with transport proteins to modulate their activity |
| Can membrane proteins alter their intracellular/extracellular face orientation? | No |
| Can membrane proteins alter their lateral orientation within the plasma membrane? | Yes |
| What factors dictate the maximum rate of facilitated diffusion? | Number of transporters, rate of channel action, affinity of the transporter for the molecule, concentration of the molecule |
| What transport proteins are responsible for the facilitated diffusion of charged molecules across a lipid membrane? | Carrier proteins (more selective, slower rate of transport) and channel proteins (less selective, faster rate of transport) |
| Define passive transport. | Movement of a molecule/ion down its respective concentration/ electrochemical gradient (requires no expenditure of energy) |
| Define active transport. | Movement of a molecule/ion against its respective concentration/ electrochemical gradient (requires expenditure of energy) |
| Which type of transport proteins can carry out active transport? | Only carrier proteins |
| Where do primary transporters allocate the energy required for active transport? | Adenosine triphosphate (ATP) hydrolysis |
| How do secondary transporters allocate the energy required for active transport? | They couple the movement of a molecule against its concentration gradient to the movement of another molecule down its concentration gradient. |

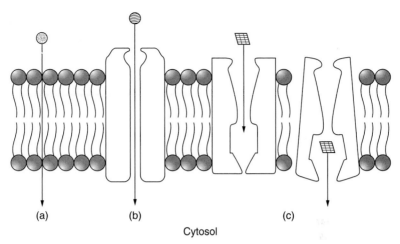

**Figure 6.3**  Channel Proteins. (a) Simple Diffusion; (b) Ion Channel-Mediated Diffusion; (c) Carrier Protein-Mediated Diffusion.

| | |
|---|---|
| Channel proteins typically transport what type of molecules? | Small, inorganic ions |
| The gating mechanism determines what functional property of a channel protein? | Permeability |
| Gating mechanisms are classified into what three categories? | Voltage-gated, ligand-gated, and mechanically-gated mechanisms |
| Carrier proteins typically transport what type of molecules? | Although more selective, they may transport any type of molecule |
| What are the four major classes of carrier proteins? | Uniporters, antiporters, symporters, ion-transporting ATPases |

## NA$^+$/K$^+$ ATPASE

| | |
|---|---|
| List some key cell functions in which maintenance of low Na$^+$ and high K$^+$ concentrations intracellularly are important. | Regulation of voltage, regulation of pH, membrane potential, transport of metabolites, water balance |
| Where in the cell is the Na$^+$/K$^+$ ATPase located? | Exclusively in the plasma membrane of all cell types (especially in neurons) |
| What is the net influx and efflux of Na$^+$ and K$^+$ per catalytic cycle? | For each ATP consumed, 3Na$^+$ leave and 2K$^+$ enter the cell |
| How many subunits does the Na$^+$/K$^+$ ATPase have? | Tetrameric; two $\alpha$-subunits which contain the binding sites for Na$^+$/K$^+$, ATP and ouabain, and two glycosylated $\beta$-subunits which play a role in maturation and localization |

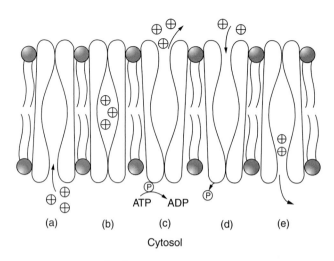

**Figure 6.4**  Na$^+$/K$^+$ ATPase. (a) 3 Na$^+$ from Cytosol into Na$^+$/K$^+$ ATPase; (b) 3 Na$^+$ inside Na$^+$/K$^+$ ATPase; (c) 3 Na$^+$ from Na$^+$/K$^+$ ATPase into Extracellular Space, ATP Degraded to ADP, Phosphate Group Binds Na$^+$/K$^+$ ATPase; (d) 2 K$^+$ from Cytosol into Na$^+$/K$^+$ ATPase, Phosphate Group Unbinds from Na$^+$/K$^+$ ATPase; (e) 2 K$^+$ from Na$^+$/K$^+$ ATPase into Cytosol.

| | |
|---|---|
| What is meant by the term electrogenic transporter? | Activity of the transporter creates an electrical current |
| What percentage of all metabolic energy in a resting organism is directed at fueling the Na$^+$/K$^+$ ATPase? | 30% |
| Describe the mechanism by which digitalis (ouabain) increases cardiac contractility. | Digitalis competes with K$^+$ for binding on the extracellular surface of the transporter. This shuts off the phosphatase activity and interrupts the phosphorylation/ dephosphorylation cycle, which leads to an increased Na$^+$ concentration intracellularly. Without a Na$^+$ concentration/electrochemical gradient, the Na$^+$/Ca$^{2+}$ antiport loses functionality and results in an increased intracellular concentration of Ca$^{2+}$. Greater intracellular Ca$^{2+}$ concentration causes stronger and longer contractions of cardiac muscle. |
| What electrolyte must the dosage of digitalis (ouabain) be controlled for? | K$^+$ |

# MAJOR ION TRANSPORT PROTEINS

List some key cell functions in which $Ca^{2+}$ plays a major role.

Contraction of all types of muscle, secretion of hormones and neurotransmitters, cell division, directed migration of nonmuscle cells, processing of visual pigments, apoptosis, and acute regulation of carbohydrate metabolism

What $Ca^{2+}$-binding protein is found in all cell types?

Calmodulin

What are the two types of $Ca^{2+}$ transport channels?

Voltage-gated and ligand-gated $Ca^{2+}$ channels

Which type of $Ca^{2+}$ channel is important in the contraction/relaxation cycle of cardiac muscle and the constriction/dilation cycle of vascular smooth muscle?

Voltage-gated $Ca^{2+}$ channels (cardiac and smooth muscle cells have slow $Ca^{2+}$ channels but skeletal muscle does not)

What drugs target the aforementioned $Ca^{2+}$ channels?

Dihydropyridine $Ca^{2+}$ blockers

Which type of $Ca^{2+}$ channel is found in the sarcoplasmic reticulum of striated muscle cells?

Ligand-gated $Ca^{2+}$ channels

Where in the cell is the $Na^+/Ca^{2+}$ antiporter located?

In the plasma membrane

What is the main role of the $Na^+/Ca^{2+}$ antiporter?

To remove excess cytosolic $Ca^{2+}$

The $Na^+/Ca^{2+}$ antiporter is ultimately dependent on what other transporter in order to function?

$Na^+/K^+$ ATPase; the $Na^+$ gradient created by the $Na^+/K^+$ ATPase produces an influx of $Na^+$ which is the driving force behind the eventual efflux of $Ca^{2+}$

List the three types of $Ca^{2+}$ ATPases along with their regulatory molecules.

Plasma membrane form (calmodulin-regulated), endoplasmic/sarcoplasmic reticulum form (not regulated), cardiac sarcoplasmic reticulum form (phospholamban-regulated)

What is the ideal intracellular pH?

7.1

Why does $H^+$ move into the cell (remember the ideal extracellular pH is 7.4)?

Negative membrane potential creates an electrochemical gradient causing $H^+$ influx

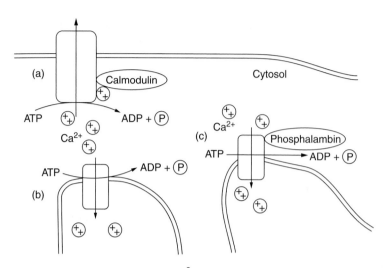

**Figure 6.5**   Three Types of $Ca^{2+}$ ATPases. (a) Plasma Membrane Form; (b) Endoplasmic/Sarcoplasmic Reticulum Form; (c) Cardiac Sarcoplasmic Reticulum Form.

| | |
|---|---|
| What are the typical pH values in subcellular organelles such as the mitochondria and lysosomes? | Mitochondrial pH is 8, lysosomal pH is 5 |
| Describe the activity of the $Na^+/H^+$ antiporter. | The influx of $Na^+$ is used to efflux $H^+$ in a 1:1 ratio |
| What activates the $Na^+/H^+$ antiporter? | Drop in pH (as in glycolysis), growth factors, protein kinase C (PKC), oncogenes |
| What inhibits the $Na^+/H^+$ antiporter? | Amiloride, cyclic adenosine monophosphate (cAMP)-dependent protein kinase |
| Why is the $Na^+$-$HCO_3^-/H^+$-$Cl^-$ exchanger twice as efficient as the $Na^+/H^+$ antiporter in alkalinizing the intracellular compartment? | Per cycle this exchanger removes $H^+$ and brings in $HCO_3^-$, which can neutralize the acidic pH |
| What drug can inhibit the $Na^+$-$HCO_3^-/H^+$-$Cl^-$ exchanger? | Stilbenedisulfonates |
| What types of cells necessary for the transport of $CO_2$ contain carbonic anhydrase? | RBCs |
| What is the major role of the $Cl^-/HCO_3^-$ exchanger? | To eliminate alkalinity in the intracellular compartment (activated when the intracellular pH rises above 7.2–7.4) |

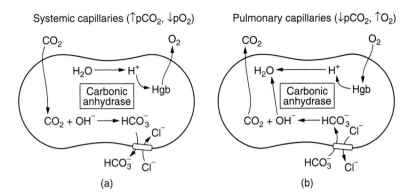

**Figure 6.6**   $CO_2$ Transport in RBCs. (a) Systemic Capillaries; (b) Pulmonary Capillaries.

| | |
|---|---|
| **What cells of the gastrointestinal (GI) tract express the $H^+$ ATPase?** | Parietal cells of the stomach |
| **What syndrome of recurrent stomach and duodenal ulcers is caused by a gastrin-secreting tumor?** | Zollinger-Ellison syndrome |
| **What class of drugs is used to treat this disorder?** | $H^+$ ATPase/proton pump inhibitors (i.e., omeprazole, lansoprazole) |
| **The $Na^+$, $K^+$, $2Cl^-$ cotransporter has the net effect of increasing the concentration of what ion intracellularly?** | $Cl^-$ |
| **Where in the nephron can the $Na^+$, $K^+$, $2Cl^-$ cotransporter be found?** | Luminal surface of the thick ascending loop of Henle (where NaCl is reabsorbed) |
| **What disorder characterized by secondary hyperaldosteronism, hypokalemic alkalosis, and growth retardation may be associated with an autosomal recessive defect in the $Na^+$, $K^+$, $2Cl^-$ cotransporter?** | Bartter syndrome |
| **What drug used to treat hypertension inhibits the $Na^+$, $K^+$, $2Cl^-$ cotransporter?** | Furosemide |
| **What factor is important in the regulation of $Cl^-$ channels?** | Concentration of other ions (i.e., $Ca^{2+}$) |
| **What protein is needed to phosphorylate, and thus activate the $Cl^-$ channel?** | Protein kinase A (PKA) |
| **What disease characterized by recurrent pulmonary infections, pancreatic insufficiency, and bronchiectasis is a result of a defective $Cl^-$ transport?** | Cystic fibrosis |

## NUCLEUS

| | |
|---|---|
| **Do eukaryotic or prokaryotic cells typically have a nucleus?** | Eukaryotic cells |
| **What cells found in the human body do not have a nucleus?** | RBCs |
| **What forms of RNA are synthesized in the nucleus?** | All forms (i.e., ribosomal RNA, messenger RNA, transfer RNA [rRNA, mRNA, tRNA]) |
| **What structures constitute the nuclear envelope?** | Two parallel membranes with an intervening perinuclear cisterna |
| **What is the fibrous protein meshwork that coats the inner nuclear membrane and plays a role in structurally organizing the nucleus?** | The nuclear lamina |
| **What is the role of a nuclear pore?** | To allow for the exchange of molecules between the nucleus and cytoplasm |
| **What nuclear inclusion is involved in the synthesis of rRNA and its assembly into ribosome precursors?** | The nucleolus |
| **In what phase of the cell cycle does the nucleolus disappear?** | Mitosis |
| **What is the main role of chromatin?** | RNA synthesis |

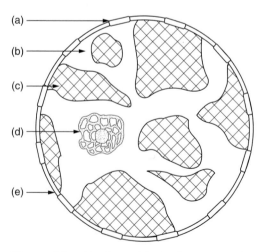

**Figure 6.7**   Nucleus. (a) Nuclear Pore; (b) Euchromatin; (c) Heterochromatin; (d) Nucleolus; (e) Nuclear Membrane.

| | |
|---|---|
| Name the two forms of chromatin. | Heterochromatin and euchromatin |
| Which form of chromatin corresponds to the Barr body in female mammalian cells? | Heterochromatin |
| Name a disorder in which no Barr body would be seen in the nucleus of a female mammalian cell. | Turner's syndrome (XO) |
| Name a disorder in which a Barr body would be seen in the nucleus of a male mammalian cell. | Klinefelter's syndrome (XXY) |
| During mitosis, what term describes division of the nucleus and of the cytoplasm? | Karyokinesis; cytokinesis |
| What form of cell division produces a haploid chromosome number? | Meiosis |

## ENDOPLASMIC RETICULUM

| | |
|---|---|
| The endoplasmic reticulum is continuous with what nuclear structure? | Outer nuclear membrane |
| The rough endoplasmic reticulum synthesizes which proteins? | Membrane-packaged proteins including secretory, plasma membrane, and lysosomal proteins |
| What molecule may be added to proteins in the rough endoplasmic reticulum? | N-linked oligosaccharides |
| List the cell types with abundant rough endoplasmic reticulum. | Mucin-secreting goblet cells, antibody-secreting plasma cells |
| Describe the role of the smooth endoplasmic reticulum. | Steroid synthesis, detoxification of drugs, muscle contraction and relaxation |
| What cell types are rich in smooth endoplasmic reticulum? | Leydig cells, adrenal cortex cells, hepatocytes, skeletal muscle cells |

## MITOCHONDRIA

| | |
|---|---|
| The outer and inner membranes subdivide mitochondria into what two compartments? | Intermembrane compartment and matrix compartment |
| Mitochondria contain what structures? | Enzymes of the tricarboxylic acid (TCA) cycle, elementary particles (including ATP synthase), circular DNA, mRNA, tRNA, rRNA |

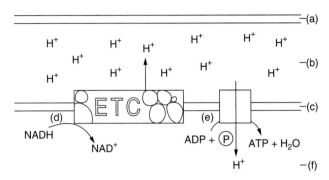

**Figure 6.8** Chemosmotic Coupling in the Electron Transport Chain. (a) Outer Mitochondrial Membrane; (b) Intermitochondrial Membrane space; (c) Inner Mitochondrial Membrane; (d) NADH Dehydrogenase; (e) Mitochondrial ATPase; (f) Mitochondrial Matrix.

| | |
|---|---|
| **What is the most important role of mitochondria?** | ATP synthesis |
| **What cells in the body do not contain mitochondria?** | RBCs |
| **Name two mechanisms by which mitochondria produce ATP.** | Via the TCA cycle (oxidation of fatty acids, amino acids, and glucose) and via the electron transport chain |
| **During electron transport, $H^+$ ions are pumped from where to where?** | $H^+$ ions are pumped from the matrix compartment across the inner mitochondrial membrane into the intermembrane compartment |
| **What substances can directly inhibit electron transport?** | Antimycin A, $CN^-$, CO, rotenone |
| **What happens to the $H^+$ gradient when electron transport is inhibited?** | Decreases because electron transport is inhibited |
| **What are possible treatments for poisoning with electron transport inhibitors?** | Supplemental $O_2$, amyl/sodium nitrate ($CN^-$ scavenger), methemoglobin |
| **By what mechanism does oligomycin poison oxidative phosphorylation?** | Directly inhibiting mitochondrial ATPase |
| **What is the effect of oligomycin on the $H^+$ gradient?** | Increases, because $H^+$ is pumped into the intermembrane compartment but it is sequestered there |
| **How does 2,4-dinitrophenylhydrazine (DNP) poison oxidative phosphorylation?** | Uncouples oxidative phosphorylation by increasing the permeability of the inner mitochondrial membrane |

| What is the effect of 2,4-DNP on the $H^+$ gradient and on $O_2$ consumption? | Decreases the $H^+$ gradient because $H^+$ pumped into the intermembrane compartment travels back into the matrix compartment without being coupled to ATP production; in order to compensate for the decreased $H^+$ gradient, electron transport continues and $O_2$ consumption is increased |
|---|---|
| What type of cell uses a mechanism similar to that of 2,4-DNP poisoning to produce heat? | Brown fat cells have a special transport protein in the inner mitochondrial membrane that uncouples respiration from ATP synthesis to produce heat |
| Mitochondrial myopathies are transmitted through which parent? | Mother (all offspring of affected females may show signs of disease) |

## GOLGI APPARATUS

| List the functions of the Golgi apparatus. | Distributing proteins and lipids |
|---|---|
| | Modifying $N$-oligosaccharides on asparagine residues |
| | Adding $O$-oligosaccharides to serine and threonine residues |
| | Assembling proteoglycans from proteoglycan core proteins |
| | Adding sulfur to sugars in proteoglycans and tyrosine residues in proteins |
| | Adding mannose-6-phosphate to specific lysosomal proteins |
| | Recycling and redistributing membranes |
| What organelle is the cis-Golgi network associated with? | Rough endoplasmic reticulum |
| How are proteins transferred to the Golgi apparatus? | Vesicles bud off from the rough endoplasmic reticulum and fuse with the cis-Golgi network |
| What is the role of the cis-Golgi network in protein processing? | Involved in protein sorting and retrieval |
| What is the role of the trans-Golgi network in protein processing? | Sorting proteins for their final destinations |
| Is protein transfer in the Golgi apparatus an energy-requiring process? | Yes, therefore it is dependent on ATP production |

**What organelle is responsible for the degradation of endocytosed material?**

Lysosome

**Describe the pathophysiology behind the inclusion vesicles associated with I-cell disease.**

Failure of mannose-6-phosphate addition to lysosomal enzymes causes these proteins to be secreted instead of being delivered to the lysosomes. Thus, lysosomes cannot degrade the contents of these vesicles.

**Name two types of coated vesicles.**

Clathrin-coated vesicles, coatamer-coated vesicles

**In which type of vesicle is a cage-like lattice formed around the vesicle?**

Clathrin-coated vesicle

**Which type of coat protein is formed by COPs?**

Coatamer

**Clathrin-coated vesicles are involved in what cellular functions?**

Receptor-mediated uptake (endocytosis) of specific molecules by the cell, signal-directed (regulated) transport of proteins from the trans-Golgi network to lysosomes or secretory granules

**Coatamer-coated vesicles are involved in what cellular processes?**

Constitutive protein transport within the cell, anterograde transport of molecules from the rough endoplasmic reticulum to the Golgi apparatus (COP I and COP II proteins), retrograde transport of molecules from the Golgi apparatus to the rough endoplasmic reticulum (COP I proteins only)

**How do lysosomes maintain their acidic pH?**

ATP-powered $H^+$ pumps in their membranes

**What role does the acidic lysosomal pH play in the recycling of vesicles?**

Aids in the uncoupling of receptors and ligands, which allows the receptors to return to the plasma membrane and ligands to move to a late endosome

**Do early or late endosomes have a more acidic pH?**

Late endosomes (pH = 5.5 versus early endosomes pH = 6)

**What proteins are found in late endosomes?**

Lysosomal hydrolases, lysosomal membrane proteins

**What constitutes a phagolysosome?**

Fusion of a phagocytic vacuole with a late endosome or lysosome

**What constitutes an autophagolysosome?**

Fusion of an autophagic vacuole (carrying cell components targeted for destruction) with a late endosome or lysosome

**What constitutes a multivesicular body?**

Fusion of an early endosome containing endocytic vesicles with a late endosome

**List the oxidative enzymes that can be found in peroxisomes.**

D-Amino acid oxidase, urate oxidase, catalase

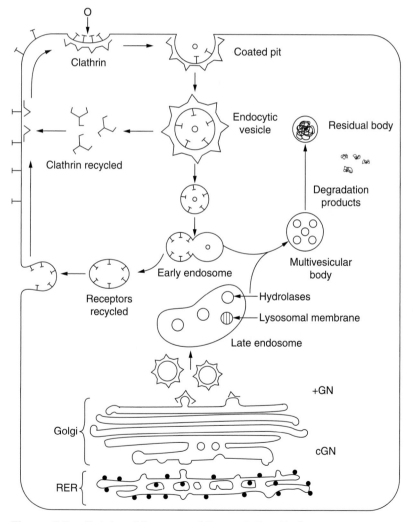

**Figure 6.9** Golgi and Lysosomal Degradation Pathway.

| | |
|---|---|
| Defective activity of what enzyme(s) can cause chronic granulomatous disease? | Nicotinamide adenosine dinucleotide phosphate (NADPH) oxidase, lysosomal lysozymes, hydrolytic enzymes |
| What test is used to confirm the diagnosis of chronic granulomatous disease? | Nitroblue tetrazolium dye reduction test (negative result confirms disease) |

## LYSOSOMAL STORAGE DISEASES

| | |
|---|---|
| What are the symptoms of Fabry's disease? | Peripheral neuropathy of the hands and feet, angiokeratomas, cardiovascular and renal disease |
| What is the deficient enzyme in Fabry's disease? | $\alpha$-Galactosidase A |
| What substrate is ultimately increased due to the enzyme deficiency in Fabry's disease? | Ceramide trihexoside (glycosphingolipid) |
| What is the inheritance pattern of Fabry's disease? | X-linked recessive |
| What are the symptoms of Krabbe's disease (globoid leukodystrophy)? | Growth retardation/difficulty feeding (remember "crabby baby"), peripheral neuropathy, hyperactive reflexes, developmental delay, and optic atrophy |
| What is the deficient enzyme in Krabbe's disease? | $\beta$-Galactosidase |
| What substrate is ultimately increased in Krabbe's disease? | Galactocerebroside |
| What is the characteristic histological finding in Krabbe's disease? | Multinucleated globoid macrophage cells |
| What is the inheritance pattern of Krabbe's disease? | Autosomal recessive |
| What are the symptoms of Gaucher disease type I? | Massive splenomegaly, *Erylenmeyer flask* bone lesions and pathologic fractures, pancytopenia, thrombocytopenia; life span is not affected |
| What are the symptoms of Gaucher disease type II? | Type II is the acute neuronopathic form; hepatosplenomegaly, central nervous system (CNS) involvement, convulsions, and mental deterioration; life span is severely affected, many dying at a young age |

| | |
|---|---|
| What is the deficient enzyme in Gaucher disease types I and II? | $\beta$-Glucocerebrosidase |
| What substrate is ultimately increased in Gaucher disease types I and II? | Glucocerebrosidase |
| What characteristic finding is seen histologically with Gaucher disease types I and II? | $p$-Aminosalicylic acid (PAS)-positive cellular inclusions |
| What inheritance pattern is seen in Gaucher disease types I and II? | Autosomal recessive |
| What are the symptoms of Niemann-Pick disease? | Delayed development, decreased visual acuity, diffuse neuronal involvement (cell death and shrinkage of the brain), massive hepatosplenomegaly, infiltration of bone marrow, death by 3 years of age |
| What is the deficient enzyme in Niemann-Pick disease? | Sphingomyelinase |
| What substrate is ultimately increased in Niemann-Pick disease? | Sphingomyelin, with build up of sphingomyelin and cholesterol in reticuloendothelial and parenchymal cells and tissues |
| What inheritance pattern is seen in Niemann-Pick disease? | Autosomal recessive |
| What sign in Niemann-Pick disease is also seen in Tay-Sachs disease? | Cherry-red spot on the macula |
| In what ethnicity is Niemann-Pick disease seen more often? | Ashkenazi Jews (similar to Tay-Sachs disease) |
| What are the symptoms of Tay-Sachs disease? | Motor and mental retardation starting at about 6 months of age, blindness, hyperacute hearing, death usually by 2–3 years of age |
| What is the deficient enzyme in Tay-Sachs disease? | Hexosaminidase A |
| What substrate is ultimately increased in Tay-Sachs disease? | $GM_2$ ganglioside |
| What characteristic findings are seen histologically with Tay-Sachs disease? | Zebra bodies |
| What inheritance pattern is seen in Tay-Sachs disease? | Autosomal recessive |
| What are the symptoms of metachromatic leukodystrophy? | Spasticity with demyelinization and gliosis, increased cerebrospinal fluid (CSF) protein, ataxia, and dementia |

| | |
|---|---|
| What is the deficient enzyme in metachromatic leukodystrophy? | Arylsulfatase A |
| What substrate is ultimately increased in metachromatic leukodystrophy? | Sulfatide, with accumulation in the brain, kidney, liver, and peripheral nerves |
| What inheritance pattern is seen in metachromatic leukodystrophy? | Autosomal recessive |
| What are the symptoms of Hurler's syndrome? | Coarse facial features (i.e., gargoylism), hepatosplenomegaly, lesions of cardiac valves, narrowing of the coronary arteries, joint stiffness, kyphoscoliosis, mental retardation, and corneal clouding |
| What is the deficient enzyme in Hurler's syndrome? | $\alpha$-L-Iduronidase |
| What substrates are ultimately increased in Hurler's syndrome? | Heparan sulfate and dermatan sulfate |
| What inheritance pattern is seen in Hurler's syndrome? | Autosomal recessive |
| What are the symptoms of Hunter's syndrome? | Mild form of Hurler's syndrome, aggressive behavior, and no corneal clouding |
| What is the deficient enzyme in Hunter's syndrome? | Iduronate sulfatase |
| What substrates are ultimately increased in Hunter's syndrome? | Heparan sulfate and dermatan sulfate |
| What inheritance pattern is seen in Hunter's syndrome? | X-linked recessive (therefore seen more in males than Hurler's) |
| Of the lysosomal storage disorders mentioned, which are inherited in an X-linked recessive pattern? | Fabry's and Hunter's syndromes |
| How are the other disorders inherited? | Autosomal recessive |

## CYTOSKELETON

| | |
|---|---|
| List the functions of the cytoskeleton. | Maintain cell shape, stabilize cell attachments, facilitate endo/exocytosis, promote cell motility |
| What are the three types of cytoskeletal filaments? | Microtubules, microfilaments, and intermediate filaments |

| | |
|---|---|
| Describe the structure of a microtubule. | Helical array of polymerized $\alpha$- and $\beta$-tubulin (13 per circumference) |
| The microtubule organizing center is also known as what structure? | Centrosome |
| During cell division, where do microtubules attach on a chromosome? | Centromere |
| What proteins aid in the polymerization of tubulin? | MAPs (microtubule-associated proteins), tau proteins |
| What disease results from impaired polymerization of tubulin in leukocytes? | Chediak-Higashi syndrome |
| Describe the pathophysiology behind the neurofibrillary tangles associated with Alzheimer's disease? | Abnormally phosphorylated tau protein |
| What drugs act on microtubules? | Mebendazole/thiabendazole (antihelminthic), taxol (antibreast cancer), colchicine (antigout), vincristine/vinblastine (anticancer), griseofulvin (antifungal) |
| What term describes the microtubule complex of flagella and cilia? | Axoneme |
| What proteins associated with microtubules are involved in neuronal axoplasmic transport? | Kinesins (anterograde) and dyneins (retrograde) |
| What protein is defective in Kartagener's syndrome? | Dynein, which leads to immotile cilia |
| Describe the structure of a microfilament. | Globular actin monomers (G-proteins) linked to a double helix |
| Microfilaments are involved with what cellular processes? | Establishing focal contact between the cell and extracellular matrix, locomotion of nonmuscle cells, formation of the contractile ring in dividing cells, folding of epithelia into tubes during development |
| Microfilaments are an important component of what GI cell structure? | Microvilli |
| What is the importance of these structures in the GI tract? | Increase the absorptive surface area |
| Name some key intermediate filaments. | Keratin, desmin, vimentin, neurofilaments, glial fibrillary acidic protein, lamins |
| What is the role of intermediate filaments? | Providing mechanical strength to cells |

| | |
|---|---|
| **What disease characterized by acantholysis with painful oral ulcers is a result of auto-antibody destruction of either desmoglein or transmembrane *E*-cadherin adhesion molecules?** | Pemphigus vulgaris |

## ORGANELLE INTERACTIONS

| | |
|---|---|
| **What term describes the uptake of materials by a cell?** | Endocytosis |
| **Describe the sequence of events occurring in receptor-mediated endocytosis.** | Ligand binds specifically to its receptor on the cell surface |
| | Ligand-receptor complex clusters into a clathrin-coated pit that invaginates and produces a clathrin-coated vesicle containing the ligand |
| | Within the cytoplasm the clathrin coat is rapidly lost, leaving an uncoated endocytic vesicle containing the ligand |
| **What genetic defects can cause familial hypercholesterolemia?** | Either the inability to synthesize low-density lipoprotein (LDL) receptors or synthesis of defective LDL receptors that cannot bind LDLs and/or clathrin-coated pits |
| **Phagocytosis is commonly a characteristic of what type of cell?** | Macrophages |
| **The aforementioned cell binds to bacteria via which of its receptors?** | Fc receptors, C3b receptors |
| **Exocytosis requires an interaction between receptors on what two cellular structures?** | The granule destined for exocytosis and the plasma membrane |
| **What are the two forms of exocytosis?** | Regulated secretion and constitutive secretion |
| **Which form of exocytosis requires an extracellular signal?** | Regulated secretion |
| **Describe the concept of membrane recycling.** | The secretory granule membrane added to the plasma membrane surface during exocytosis is retrieved during endocytosis via the clathrin-coated vesicles. Thus, the surface area of the plasma membrane remains relatively constant. |

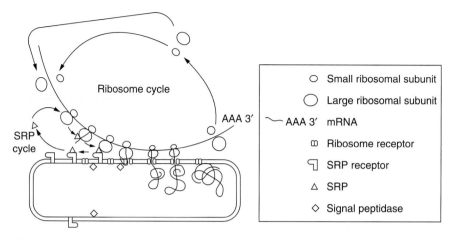

**Figure 6.10**   Signal Hypothesis.

**Where in the cell are ribosomes, which synthesize membrane-packaged proteins, located?**

On the surface of the rough endoplasmic reticulum (RER)

**Where are free signal recognition particles (SRPs) found in the cell?**

Cytoplasm

**SRPs bind to what portion of the ribosome-mRNA complex?**

Signal sequence of mRNA

**What structures anchor the polyribosomes-mRNA-SRP complex to the RER membrane following relocation of this complex from the cytosol to the RER?**

Ribosome receptor proteins and SRP receptors in the RER membrane

**Newly formed polypeptide is threaded through what structure in the RER membrane?**

A pore across the RER membrane (thus, the polypeptide is pushed into the RER cisterna)

**What happens to the newly synthesized polypeptide once in the RER cisterna?**

Signal peptidase cleaves the SRP, polypeptide is glycosylated

**Newly synthesized polypeptide is transferred next from the RER cisterna to what organelle?**

cis-Golgi network (via coatamer-coated vesicles)

**In what direction do proteins destined for membrane packing move in the Golgi apparatus?**

From the cis to the trans face of the Golgi apparatus (again via coatamer-coated vesicles)

**Do all of the events of protein processing occur in the same compartment of the Golgi apparatus?**

No, they occur in distinct cisternal subcompartments

**What part of the Golgi apparatus sorts proteins for their final destinations?**

trans-Golgi network

## CELL-TO-CELL COMMUNICATION

| | |
|---|---|
| Name some examples of signaling molecules. | Neurotransmitters, endocrine hormones, local mediators (paracrine hormones, autocrine hormones), $Ca^{2+}$ ions (intracellularly) |
| What are the two classes of signaling molecules? | Lipid-soluble signaling molecules<br>Hydrophilic-signaling molecules |
| Where does each of these classes of signaling molecules bind in the cell? | Lipid-soluble molecules penetrate the plasma membrane and bind receptors in the cytoplasm or nucleus<br>Hydrophilic molecules bind cell surface receptors |
| How does each class of signaling molecules create an effect in a cell? | Lipid-soluble molecule-receptor complexes interact directly with DNA-binding sites (therefore creating slow-acting, long-term effects)<br>Hydrophilic molecule-receptor complexes are coupled to second messenger systems and phosphorylation of cellular proteins (therefore creating fast-acting, short-term effects) |

## RECEPTORS

| | |
|---|---|
| What signaling molecules utilize intracellular receptors? | Progesterone, estrogen, testosterone, cortisol, aldosterone, thyroxine (remember PET CAT) |
| Nuclear hormone receptor complexes bind to DNA and stimulate what enzymatic modification of histones? | Acetyl transferase acetylates histones resulting in opening/relaxation of DNA |
| What amino acid residues compose the DNA-binding regions of steroid hormone receptors? | Cysteine residues |
| What disorder is characterized by hypertension, truncal obesity, hyperglycemia, buffalo hump, and immune suppression? | Cushing's syndrome |
| What glucocorticoid/progesterone receptor inhibitor has been used to treat the aforementioned disorder, and recently as an abortion method? | Mifepristone (RU486) |

| | |
|---|---|
| **What receptor gates the Na⁺/K⁺ ion channel?** | Nicotinic acetylcholine receptor |
| **Antibodies to this receptor results in what disease?** | Myasthenia gravis |
| **What drug can be used to treat this disease?** | Neostigmine (acetylcholine esterase inhibitor) |
| **What signaling molecules utilize the receptor tyrosine kinase (RTK)?** | Insulin, epidermal growth factor, platelet-derived growth factor |
| **Describe the chain of events leading to activation of the RTK.** | Ligand binds the extracellular domain of the RTK |
| | RTK dimerizes with the adjacent RTK |
| | Intracellular kinase domains activated |
| | Intracellular autophosphorylation of the RTK |
| | Phosphorylated residues become the recognition/anchoring sites for other RTK substrates |
| **The signal termination of RTK is accomplished via what mechanism?** | Internalization of the RTK-signaling molecule complex into an endosome |
| **What disease can be caused by either a decrease in the number of insulin receptors or a dysfunction in the signaling of insulin receptors?** | Type II diabetes mellitus |

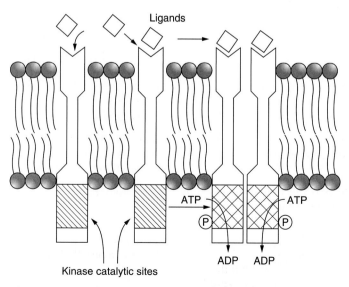

**Figure 6.11**  Ligand-Induced Conformation States of RTK.

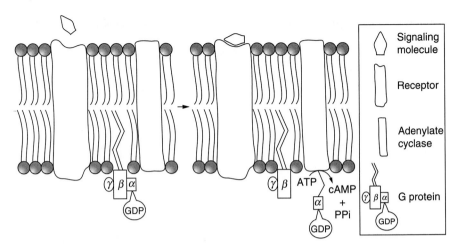

**Figure 6.12** Functioning of GPRs.

| | |
|---|---|
| **What class of drugs increases the target cell receptors' response to insulin?** | Glitazones (pioglitazone, rosiglitazone, troglitazone) |
| **What signaling molecules utilize G-protein-coupled receptors (GPRs)?** | Catecholamines, hormones, local mediators |
| **Describe the chain of events following binding of the signaling molecule to the $G_s$PR.** | Signaling molecule binds to the receptor |
| | $\alpha$-Subunit of the $G_s$ protein binds guanosine 5'-triphosphate (GTP), dissociating from the $\beta$- and $\gamma$-subunits |
| | GTP-$\alpha$-subunit complex activates adenylate cyclase |
| | cAMP produced from ATP |
| | cAMP activates PKA (cAMP-dependent PKA) |
| **List the $G_s$PRs.** | $\beta_1$, $\beta_2$, $D_1$, $H_2$, $V_2$ |
| **What bacteria elaborate toxins that constitutively activate the GPR?** | *Bordatella pertussis* or *Vibrio cholera*, via adenosine diphosphate (ADP) ribosylation of the $\alpha$-subunit |
| **Cellular cAMP levels can be increased by inhibiting what enzyme?** | Phosphodiesterase |
| **Name some inhibitors of the aforementioned enzyme.** | Caffeine, sildenafil, tadalafil, milrinone, theophylline |
| **What effect do $G_i$PRs have on cAMP production?** | Decrease cAMP production by inhibiting adenylate cyclase |

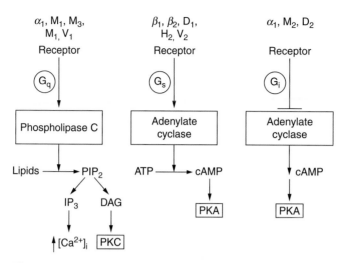

**Figure 6.13** GPR-Linked Second Messengers Diagram.

| | |
|---|---|
| List the $G_i$PRs. | $\alpha_2$, $M_2$, $D_2$ |
| What enzyme is activated following binding of the signaling molecule to the $G_q$PR? | Phospholipase C, leading to formation of inositol triphosphate and diacylglycerol |
| What are the eventual effectors following $G_q$PR activation? | Increased intracellular $Ca^{2+}$, activation of PKC |
| List the $G_q$PRs. | $\alpha_1$, $M_1$, $M_3$, $H_1$, $V_1$ |

## ARACHIDONIC ACID PRODUCTS

| | |
|---|---|
| What enzyme liberates arachidonic acid from the plasma membrane? | Phospholipase $A_2$ |
| Name an inhibitor of this enzyme. | Corticosteroids (halobetasol, hydrocortisone, dexamethasone, prednisone) |
| What toxicity is associated with this inhibitor? | Iatrogenic Cushing's syndrome—truncal obesity, moon facies, buffalo hump, muscle wasting, osteoporosis, easy bruisability |
| What enzyme is responsible for hydroperoxide (i.e., leukotriene) production from arachidonic acid? | Lipooxygenase |
| Name an inhibitor of this enzyme. | Zileuton |

| | |
|---|---|
| **List the hydroperoxides and their functions.** | LT $B_4$ is a neutrophil chemotactic agent; LT $C_4$, $D_4$, and $E_4$ function in bronchoconstriction, vasoconstriction, contraction of smooth muscle, and increasing vascular permeability |
| **What drugs inhibit hydroperoxide function?** | Zafirlukast, montelukast |
| **What enzyme is responsible for endoperoxide (i.e., thromboxane, prostaglandin, and prostacyclin) production from arachidonic acid?** | Cyclooxygenase (COX-1, COX-2) |
| **Name the inhibitors of this enzyme.** | Aspirin (irreversibly inhibits COX-1 and COX-2), nonsteroidal anti-inflammatory drugs (NSAIDs) (reversibly inhibit COX-1 and COX-2), celecoxib/rofecoxib (inhibits COX-2 only), acetaminophen (reversibly inhibits COX-1 and COX-2, mostly in the CNS) |

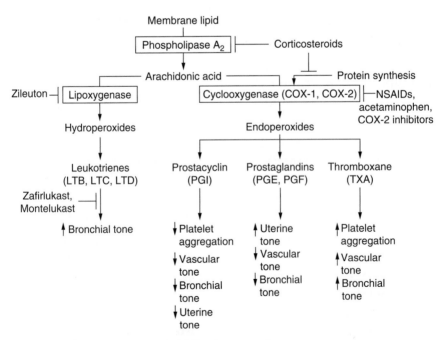

**Figure 6.14**  Arachidonic Acid Products.

List the endoperoxides and their functions. | Thromboxane $A_2$ (Tx$A_2$) stimulates platelet aggregation and vasoconstriction; prostaglandin E (PGE) and prostaglandin F (PGF) increase uterine tone and stimulate vasodilation and bronchodilation; prostaglandin I (PGI) inhibits platelet aggregation, decreases uterine tone, and stimulates vasodilation and bronchodilation

## MUSCLE

| | |
|---|---|
| What is a neuromuscular junction? | Synapse between a nerve and a muscle cell |
| What neurotransmitter is typically found in a neuromuscular junction? | Acetylcholine |
| What toxin prevents exocytosis of secretory vesicles containing this neurotransmitter? | Botulinum toxin (causing flaccid paralysis) |
| What toxin blocks inhibition of neurotransmitter release? | Tetanus toxin (causing tetanic paralysis) |
| Name one depolarizing and one nondepolarizing neuromuscular blocking agent. | Succinylcholine (depolarizing), tubocurarine (nondepolarizing) |
| Name the connective tissue layer which contains the blood supply to skeletal muscle. | Endomysium |
| What connective tissue layer surrounds individual skeletal muscle fibers? | Perimysium |
| What connective tissue layer surrounds the bundles of skeletal muscle fibers? | Epimysium |
| What is a myofiber? | A single multinucleated muscle cell |
| What are regularly arranged filaments of myofiber termed? | Myofibrils |
| Describe the boundaries of a sarcomere in the myofiber. | Region between two Z disks |
| What is the function of the Z disk? | Anchor thin filaments to the sarcomere |
| What protein composes | |
|     Thick filaments? | Myosin |
|     Thin filaments? | Actin |

| | |
|---|---|
| Name the area of the myofiber that contains the thick filaments and stains dark. | A-band |
| Name the area of the myofiber within the A-band that stains lighter. | H-band |
| Name the area of the myofiber that contains the thin filaments and stains light. | I-band |
| What is a T-tubule? | The transverse tubule that passes from the sarcolemma across a myofibril |
| What is the sarcoplasmic reticulum? | Muscle endoplasmic reticulum containing $Ca^{2+}$ ion stores |
| What is a dihydropyridine receptor? | A voltage-gated receptor located on the plasma membrane of a muscle cell that acts as $Ca^{2+}$ channel |
| What is a ryanodine receptor? | A voltage-gated receptor located on the muscle endoplasmic reticulum that acts as a $Ca^{2+}$ channel |
| What disorder is characterized by excessive $Ca^{2+}$ release from the sarcoplasmic reticulum? | Malignant hyperthermia (result of abnormal opening of the ryanodine receptor) |
| What drug is used to treat this disorder? | Dantrolene |
| Describe the sequence of events leading to skeletal muscle contraction following the binding of acetylcholine to the acetylcholine receptor. | Depolarization travels down the T-tubule |
| | The dihydropyridine receptor activates the ryanodine receptor to release $Ca^{2+}$ |
| | Released $Ca^{2+}$ binds troponin C |
| | Troponin C changes conformation |
| | Tropomyosin moves out of the myosin-binding groove on the actin filament |
| | Myosin hydrolyzes its bound ATP and is displaced on the actin filament (power stroke) |
| | Contraction causes HIZ shrinkage |
| What protein anchors the cortical cytoskeleton of a muscle cell to the transmembrane glycoproteins? | Dystrophin |
| What disease manifests as a result of a defect in the aforementioned protein? | Duchenne's muscular dystrophy |
| What structures physically connect cardiac muscle cells? | Intercalated discs |

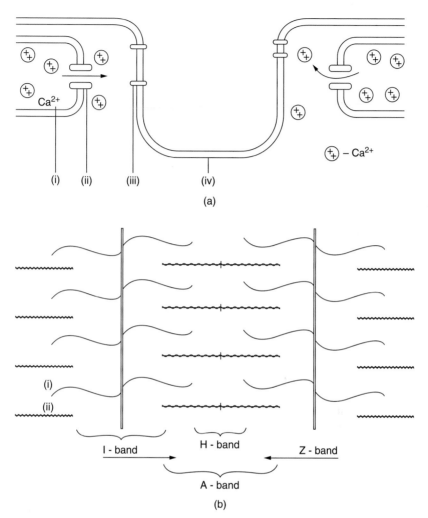

**Figure 6.15** Skeletal Muscle Contraction. (a) Sarcoplasmic Reticulum:
(i) Sarcoplasmic Reticulum, (ii) Ryanodine Receptor, (iii) Dihydropyridine
Receptor, (iv) T-Tubule Membrane; (b) HIZ Shrinkage: (i) Actin Thin
Filament, (ii) Myosin Thick Filament.

| | |
|---|---|
| **What structures electrically couple cardiac muscle cells?** | Gap junctions |
| **What is meant by the term *calcium-triggered calcium release* in regards to cardiac muscle cell contraction?** | Contraction is dependent on extracellular $Ca^{2+}$, which enters the cells during the plateau of an action potential and stimulates the release of sequestered $Ca^{2+}$ from the sarcoplasmic reticulum |

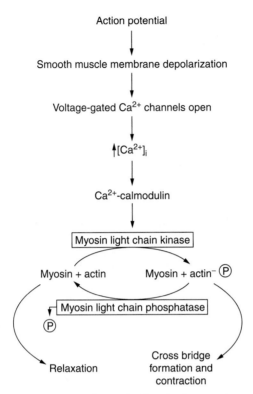

Action potential

Smooth muscle membrane depolarization

Voltage-gated $Ca^{2+}$ channels open

$\uparrow[Ca^{2+}]_i$

$Ca^{2+}$-calmodulin

Myosin light chain kinase

Myosin + actin      Myosin + actin$^-$ Ⓟ

Myosin light chain phosphatase

Ⓟ

Relaxation          Cross bridge formation and contraction

**Figure 6.16**  Smooth Muscle Contraction.

| | |
|---|---|
| **What two proteins remove excess $Ca^{2+}$ from the cytoplasm of a cardiac muscle cell following a contraction cycle?** | $Ca^{2+}$-ATPase and $Na^+/Ca^{2+}$ exchanger |
| **What drug is used to increase cardiac contractility indirectly by inhibiting the removal of excess $Ca^{2+}$?** | Digitalis (ouabain) |
| **What ion-protein complex activates myosin light chain kinase in smooth muscle cells?** | $Ca^{2+}$-calmodulin |
| **Does myosin light chain kinase activation result in contraction or relaxation?** | Contraction |
| **Increased intracellular levels of what second messenger will typically result in smooth muscle relaxation?** | Cyclic guanosine monophosphate (cGMP) |
| **What drug used to treat male impotence reduces breakdown of the aforementioned second messenger?** | Viagra (cGMP phosphodiesterase inhibitor) |
| **What drug used to treat severe hypertension reduces afterload?** | Hydralazine (vasodilates arterioles > veins) |

# CHAPTER 7

# Vignettes

A 43-year-old African-American man arrives at the emergency room with his son confused, short of breath, and smelling grossly of alcohol. Additionally, his gait showcases a significant foot drop. The son reports that the father's diet consists mainly of snacks and canned foods when he is not drinking alcohol. The son also reports the father's tendency to make up elaborate stories when discussing himself. Physical examination reveals significant hepatomegaly and decreased deep tendon reflexes. Chest x-ray (CXR) shows cardiomegaly with basal lung congestion.

| | |
|---|---|
| What vitamin may be deficient in this patient? | Thiamine, vitamin $B_1$ |
| The cardiac failure and polyneuropathy encountered are manifestations of which disease? | Wet beriberi and dry beriberi, respectively |
| In what order should deficient nutrients be administered to this patient? | Thiamine first, followed by glucose, folate, and other vitamins |

A 39-year-old alcoholic man reports the insidious onset of "not feeling like himself" and "forgetting things." His review of systems is significant for the coinciding appearance of chronic diarrhea. He reports that his diet consists of many wheat and corn products. The physical examination is significant for an erythematous, nonpruitic, hyperpigmented, scaling rash of the face, neck, and dorsum of the hands.

| | |
|---|---|
| The constellation of signs and symptoms suggests what disease? | Pellegra |
| This disease is a result of what vitamin deficiency? | Niacin, vitamin $B_3$ |
| What is the treatment of choice? | Oral nicotinamide |

A 17-month-old boy is brought to his pediatrician by his parents for concern regarding abnormal outward bowing of his lower extremities. In addition, the child exhibits lineal chest depression along the diaphragm, and enlargement of the costochondral junctions. The child's diet is deficient in dairy products and he spends a lot of his time playing indoors.

| | |
|---|---|
| This child is suffering from what disease? | Rickets |

| | |
|---|---|
| What would you expect this child's serum calcium, serum phosphorous, and alkaline phosphatase levels to be? | Normal/slightly low, decreased, and increased, respectively |
| What are potential treatments for this child's condition? | Increase egg and dairy product intake, increase exposure to sunlight |

A 42-year-old man who recently emigrated from Sudan sustains a femoral neck fracture when he accidentally slips in the shower. He reports that the fall was not too severe. He has been suffering from recurrent lower back pain and leg weakness.

| | |
|---|---|
| A lumbar-sacral spine x-ray would most likely show what findings? | Collapse of lumbar vertebrae and generalized osteopenia |
| This man is suffering from what condition? | Osteomalacia |
| What are potential etiologies for this man's condition? | Lack of sunlight exposure, intestinal malabsorption, renal insufficiency, target organ resistance |

A 9-month-old girl with poor perinatal care is brought to the pediatrician because of listlessness, pallor, and anorexia. The child's gums bleed easily and she has petechiae over her nasal and oral mucosa. Her coagulation tests reveal a prolonged bleeding time.

| | |
|---|---|
| What nutrient could this child be lacking in her diet? | Ascorbic acid, vitamin C |
| What role does this nutrient play in collagen formation? | Ascorbic acid hydroxylates praline and lysine |
| What other populations are at risk for developing this condition? | Smokers, oncologic patients, alcoholics, elderly |

A 33-year-old Mexican immigrant is seen in the emergency department after crashing his taxi cab late that night. He claims to not have suffered any major injuries but does mention that his visual acuity at night has decreased significantly since he arrived in the United States 3 years ago.

| | |
|---|---|
| What physical signs can you look for to confirm this man's condition? | Conjunctival xerosis, Bitot's spots |
| This man's diet is deficient for what vitamin? | Retinol, vitamin A |
| How is this vitamin involved in visual acuity? | Retinol is used for the synthesis of rhodopsin in the retina |

An elderly appearing alcoholic man with a history of seizures comes to the emergency room with hematemesis, hemarthrosis of his left knee, bleeding gums, and generalized weakness. The man reports that he takes phenytoin as an antiepileptic medication. Physical examination reveals a thin and malnourished man with subcutaneous ecchymosis in his arms and legs. Coagulation tests show a prolonged prothrombin time (PT) and partial thromboplastin time (PTT).

| | |
|---|---|
| This man's presentation is consistent with deficiency of which vitamin? | Vitamin K |
| Which coagulation factors are dependent upon this vitamin for their activity? | Factors II, VII, IX, and X (via $\gamma$-carboxylation) |
| What other situations can predispose to this type of bleeding? | Broad-spectrum antibiotic use, malabsorption, dietary vitamin K deficiency |

A 27-year-old woman presents to her physician with weakness, easy fatigability, nausea, and diarrhea but no neurological signs. She reports that she does not regularly eat green leafy vegetables. A complete blood count (CBC) shows hypersegmented polymorphonuclear neutrophils (PMNs) and a megaloblastic anemia.

| | |
|---|---|
| This woman's diet is likely deficient in which nutrient? | Folate |
| What is the importance of this nutrient? | Folate is used in the synthesis of DNA and RNA; it also acts as a coenzyme for one-carbon transfer and is involved in methylation reactions |
| If this woman becomes pregnant, her fetus would be at risk for what congenital abnormalities? | Neural tube defects |

A 32-year-old White male is recovering from what was properly diagnosed as an acute myocardial infarction the previous day. Physical examination reveals xanthelasmas, arcus senilis, and painful xanthomas of the Achilles tendon and patellae. The man's father died before he was 40 years of age of a myocardial infarction. Serum levels of low-density lipoprotein (LDL) are extremely high.

| | |
|---|---|
| This patient likely suffers from what disorder? | Type II hyperlipoproteinemia; familial hypercholesterolemia |
| What is the inheritance pattern of this disorder? | Autosomal dominant |
| What are the potential treatments of this disorder? | Meticulous dieting, cholesterol-lowering drugs |

A 17-year-old White female complains of midepigastric pain and nausea after eating fried foods. She also has an older sibling who suffers from the same symptoms. Her face, scalp, elbows, and knees have nonpainful, yellowish papules and she has marked hepatosplenomegaly. Labs reveal very high triglyceride levels and moderate elevation of serum cholesterol and phospholipids.

| | |
|---|---|
| This girl's complaints and family history are suggestive of what diagnosis? | Familial hypertriglyceridemia (autosomal dominant) |
| What additional markers may be elevated in this girl? | Serum amylase and lipase (recurrent acute pancreatitis) |
| What are potential treatments of this disorder? | Low-fat diet, exercise, avoidance of alcohol |

A 21-year-old gentleman is being evaluated for progressive muscle weakness. He is unable to raise his arms above his shoulders and anytime he stands for longer than 2 hours, he experiences severe pain in his legs. Electromyogram (EMG) studies were unrevealing and so a muscle biopsy done, which reveals extensive accumulation of membrane-bound glycogen along with absence of myofilaments and sarcoplasmic organelles.

| | |
|---|---|
| This patient is likely deficient in what enzyme? | $\alpha$-1,4 glucosidase (Pompe's disease) |
| Which organs are most significantly involved? | Heart and skeletal muscle |
| Diagnosis can be confirmed by what? | Enzyme assay on leukocytes or fibroblasts |

A 9 month old is seen by her pediatrician and is noted to have psychomotor retardation along with a palpable liver and spleen. Ophthalmologic examination revealed a cherry-red spot in the macula. Pulmonary and cardiac examinations were unremarkable. Bone marrow examination revealed the presence of numerous foam cells.

| | |
|---|---|
| This patient has what disease? | Niemann-Pick disease |
| This disorder particularly affects which ethnic group? | Ashkenazi Jews |
| Death usually results from what? | Neurological damage |

A 3-year-old boy is being evaluated for recurrent infections. He is found to be leukopenic and has megaloblastic hypochromic anemia. He is also noted for developmental retardation. Over the next couple of months, his anemia is found to be unresponsive to iron, folic acid, or $B_{12}$. High levels of orotic acid are found in his urine.

| | |
|---|---|
| What metabolic defect could cause this? | A defect in pyrimidine metabolism |

| | |
|---|---|
| The inheritance pattern of this disease is what? | Autosomal recessive |
| What is a possible treatment for this disease? | High-dose oral uridine |

A 6-month-old baby boy of Ashkenazi Jewish decent is evaluated by a pediatrician because of loss of motor skills and decreased attentiveness. Upon physical examination, the baby is found to have hyperreflexia with sustained ankle clonus. His liver and spleen were not palpable. Ophthalmologic examination revealed a cherry-red spot in the macula. Serum enzyme analysis reveals the absence of detectable activity in hexosaminidase A.

| | |
|---|---|
| This enzyme degrades what substance? | Ganglioside $GM_2$ |
| Intracellular accumulations occur in which cytoplasmic organelle? | Lysosome |
| Histological examination would reveal what characteristic finding in nerve cells? | Fat droplets |

A 2-month-old girl is brought to the emergency room because her mother had difficulty awakening her from an overnight sleep. The baby is found to be extremely lethargic. Laboratory workup reveals a very low blood glucose level and elevated lactate with a large anion gap. Glucagon administration produced a marked increase in lactate without hyperglycemia. Physical examination revealed a markedly enlarged liver and nonpalpable spleen.

| | |
|---|---|
| This patient is deficient in what enzyme? | Glucose-6-phosphatase (von Gierke disease) |
| Besides hypoglycemia, what is another metabolic consequence of this disease? | Hyperlipidemia |
| How can this disease be treated? | Nasogastric feeding to maintain glucose levels for infants, raw cornstarch can be used for older children |

A 40-year-old Caucasian gentleman is admitted with a hematocrit of 14. He is noted to have a lemon-yellow waxy pallor and a painful swollen beefy tongue. Neurological examination revealed paresthesias, weakness, and an unsteady gait. A peripheral blood smear shows a macrocytic anemia. Mean corpuscular volume (MCV) and mean cell hemoglobin (MCH) are increased with normal mean corpuscular hemoglobin volume (MCHV).

| | |
|---|---|
| This patient is suffering from what? | Pernicious anemia |
| This disease is characterized by a lack of what in gastric secretions? | Intrinsic factor |
| The above is used for the absorption of what? | Vitamin $B_{12}$ |

A 6-year-old Caucasian male is being evaluated for anemia. Past medical history was significant for severe jaundice and anemia at birth which was treated with an exchange transfusion. Physical examination revealed mild splenomegaly. Hemoglobin electrophoresis revealed normal hemoglobin. Erythrocyte osmotic fragility was normal and the Coombs' test was negative.

| | |
|---|---|
| What enzyme deficiency could cause this? | Pyruvate kinase deficiency |
| Patients are usually asymptomatic in nonsevere forms. What could cause symptoms in nonsevere forms? | Aplastic crisis |
| What viral infection is associated with the above? | Parvovirus B19 |

A 55-year-old man is seen in the emergency room complaining of severe pain in his right first metatarsophalangeal joint. He reports binge drinking after a fight with his wife earlier that day. His great toe is very painful to active and passive motion. In addition, physical examination reveals a lump under the skin on his left ear and olecranon bursitis.

| | |
|---|---|
| This patient is likely suffering from what disorder? | Gout |
| What would be expected to be seen on aspiration of the synovial fluid in the involved joint? | Negatively birefringent, needle-shaped crystals of uric acid salts |
| What are potential acute and long-term treatments of this disorder? | Colchicine and nonsteroidal anti-inflammatory drugs (NSAIDs) acutely; allopurinol and probenecid long term |

A 20-year-old college student presents in the emergency room seemingly confused with complaints of abdominal pain, diarrhea, and vomiting. While she is talking, a peculiar fruity breath smell is noted. She reports tailgating all day and being intoxicated following a party earlier that night. She cannot remember whether she had taken her diabetes medication.

| | |
|---|---|
| This patient is most likely what type of diabetic? | Insulin-dependent diabetes mellitus, type I, juvenile onset |
| How would her glucose, bicarbonate, and anion gap levels be changed? | Increased glucose, decreased bicarbonate, increased anion gap |
| What is the proper order of treatment? | Correction of fluid deficit if dehydrated, potassium administration, gradual lowering of glucose with insulin |

A 2-year-old is brought to the pediatrician for a well-child visit. The child is noted to have white hair, including eyelashes and eyebrows. Her skin is very pale throughout and eye examination reveals poor development of the macula with irises and pupils. The child's father has many of the same characteristics.

| This child is suffering from what disorder? | Albinism (absence of tyrosinase) |
|---|---|
| The absent enzyme catalyzes what reaction? | Tyrosinase catalyzes the conversion of tyrosine to dihydroxyphenylalanine and melanin |
| The child may be at risk for developing what skin disease? | Squamous cell cancer |

A 35-year-old man presents with dark, blackened spots in his sclera and ear cartilage. He also reports back pain and swelling of his knees. He has noticed that when he leaves his urine standing, it turns black.

| This man is suffering from what disorder? | Ochronosis, alkaptonuria |
|---|---|
| What enzyme is deficient in this condition? | Homogentisate oxidase |
| What substance would be expected to be elevated in his urine? | Homogentisic acid |

A thin-appearing 3-year-old White girl is brought by her parents to the pediatrician's office because of constant difficulty breathing. She has a consistent cough that is productive of green sputum and causes difficulty sleeping. The parents note that the child has had foul-smelling stool since birth. The child has had frequent urinary tract infections.

| The child likely is showing signs of what underlying disease? | Cystic fibrosis |
|---|---|
| How is this disease inherited? | Autosomal recessive |
| What test is routinely used to screen for this disease? | Chloride sweat test |

A 32-year-old man presents in the emergency room in acute distress with severe, intermittent left-flank pain, nausea, vomiting, and hematuria. He reports having experienced these episodes several times before. During physical examination, the man is constantly switching positions in the bed. There is prominent left costovertebral angle tenderness. Labs revealed hexagonal crystals upon cooling of acidified urine sediment.

| This patient is suffering from what disorder? | Cystinuria |
|---|---|

| | |
|---|---|
| **What is the etiology behind this condition?** | Impaired renal tubular absorption of dibasic amino acids (cysteine, ornithine, arginine, lysine) leading to increased urinary excretion and kidney stone formation |
| **What are potential treatments of this disorder?** | Low-methionine diet, increased fluid intake, urine alkalization |

A 4-year-old White male is brought by his parents to the pediatric clinic because of easy fatigability and difficulty walking of several months' duration. Concurrently, the child's calves have increased in size. The mother reports that the child has begun to "climb on himself" to rise from a sitting position.

| | |
|---|---|
| **This child likely has what disease?** | Duchenne's muscular dystrophy |
| **The child inherited his defective gene from which parent?** | The mother (X-linked recessive disorder) |
| **The disease is characterized by marked deficiency of what protein?** | Dystrophin (stabilizes actin filaments in the muscle) |

A 13-year-old boy is brought into the emergency room by his father after he dislocated his right shoulder playing rough with his little brother. Upon further questioning, it is discovered that the child has dislocated his right shoulder five times before and his left shoulder four times. He also has a history of easy bruising.

| | |
|---|---|
| **What disorder could this patient be suffering from?** | Ehlers-Danlos syndrome (cutis hyperelastica) |
| **What is the etiology of this disorder?** | Faulty collagen synthesis |
| **What other physical findings would be expected to be found?** | Hyperelastic skin, hyperextensibility of joints, blue sclera |

An 11-year-old Black girl is brought to her pediatrician's office with complaints of easy fatigability, pallor, and recurrent episodes of abdominal and chest pain. The parents are immigrants from a region of Kenya known to be endemic for malaria.

| | |
|---|---|
| **This patient may be suffering from what hemoglobinopathy?** | Sickle cell anemia |
| **What is the gene mutation found in this disorder?** | Valine substitutes glutamic acid at position 6 on the $\beta$-globin DNA chain of hemoglobin |
| **Treatment with what substance may help increase fetal hemoglobin levels?** | Hydroxyurea |

A 2-year-old male child of Greek immigrants is brought to the pediatric clinic due to marked pallor, delayed developmental motor milestone attainment, and failure to thrive. The child is noted to have mild icterus, splenomegaly, and maxillary hypertrophy. Labs reveal target cells and acanthocytes.

| | |
|---|---|
| This child is likely suffering from what blood disorder? | Thalassemia |
| What are likely the relative levels of hemoglobin A, hemoglobin A2, and hemoglobin F as compared to a normal child? | Decreased hemoglobin A, increased hemoglobin A2, increased hemoglobin F |
| What characteristic findings are expected on x-ray of the skull? | Marrow overgrowth in the maxilla, widening of diploic spaces with a "hair-on-end" appearance |

A 32-year-old male complains of diminishing vision of his left eye. Additionally, he reports painful, burning sensations of his palms and soles. His family history is significant for chronic renal failure. Physical examination reveals angiokeratomas present on the skin around his umbilicus, buttocks, and scrotum. There is a corneal leukomatous opacity and retinal edema in the left eye. There is edema in the lower extremities.

| | |
|---|---|
| What disease is this patient suffering from? | Fabry's disease |
| What is the etiology behind this disease? | X-linked recessive disorder of glycosphingolipid metabolism caused by a deficiency of $\alpha$-galactosidase A |
| What is a potentially fatal complication of this disease? | Renal failure |

An 8-week-old White male is brought into the pediatrician's office because of lethargy, difficulty feeding, occasional vomiting, and yellowing of the skin. The patient is growing in the fifth percentile. On physical examination, the patient shows irritability, jaundice, hepatomegaly, and bilateral cataracts. Urine analysis shows galactosuria.

| | |
|---|---|
| This patient is likely suffering from what disorder? | Galactosemia |
| What enzyme is deficient in this patient? | Galactose-1-phosphate uridyl transferase |
| Which organs are most severely affected by this disorder? | Liver, eyes, and brain (deposition of galactose-1-phosphate and galactitol) |

A 21-year-old mentally retarded Jewish male presents to his primary care provider with complaints of recurrent epistaxis and easy bruising. Directed questioning reveals weakness and an enlarging left-sided abdominal mass. Physical examination reveals multiple purpuric patches, pallor, mild hepatomegaly, and massive splenomegaly. Bone marrow biopsy shows "wrinkled paper" intracytoplasmic inclusions that stain $p$-aminosalicylic acid (PAS) positive.

| | |
|---|---|
| This patient has been suffering from what disorder? | Gaucher disease |
| What is the deficient enzyme and mode of inheritance of this disorder? | Glucocerebrosidase, autosomal recessive |
| What do the "wrinkled paper" inclusions represent? | Glucocerebroside deposition |

A 6-month-old baby is brought to her pediatrician because the parents have noticed frequent nausea, vomiting, and lethargy following the addition of fruit juices to the baby's previous diet of only breast milk. Labs reveal hypoglycemia with fructosemia and the baby's urine is positive for reducing sugars.

| | |
|---|---|
| What enzyme is deficient in this baby? | Aldolase b (hereditary fructose intolerance) |
| If untreated, this disease may lead to what complication? | Liver cirrhosis |
| What is the treatment for this disease? | Avoiding fructose in the diet (i.e., fruit juices, fruits, sweets) |

An 8-year-old male is referred to your pediatric specialty service because of progressive mental retardation, diminished visual acuity, and a "bird chest." Physical examination reveals long fingers and lenticular dislocation. Urine analysis shows increased urinary homocystine.

| | |
|---|---|
| This child is suffering from what disorder? | Homocystinuria |
| What are the other systemic manifestations of this disorder? | Osteoporosis, thromboses |
| How is this disorder treated? | Methionine-restricted diet, supplemental cysteine, and folate |

A 9-year-old male with a course face and large tongue is brought into the clinic because of decreased hearing. Physical examination reveals no corneal opacities. Urine analysis shows increased heparin sulfate and dermatan sulfate.

| | |
|---|---|
| What is the disease and etiology of the disorder this child suffers from? | X-linked recessive Hunter's disease (type II mucopolysaccharidosis), iduronosulfate sulfatase deficiency |

| Leukocytes will likely show what distinguishing characteristic with microscopic analysis? | Reilly bodies (metachromatic granules) |
| What auditory complication is associated with this disorder? | Deafness |

A 20-month-old mentally and physically delayed male presents with bilateral corneal clouding. The child showcases *gargoylism* with coarse, elongated facial features. Physical examination reveals cardiomegaly, hepatomegaly, and kyphoscoliosis.

| This child suffers from a deficiency of what enzyme? | $\alpha$-Iduronidase (Hurler's syndrome, type I mucopolysaccharidosis) |
| What is the mode of inheritance of this disorder? | Autosomal recessive |
| What abnormal substances would be found in this patient's urine? | Chondroitin sulfate B, heparin sulfate |

A 6-month-old infant is brought to the clinic because of failure to thrive. The mother reports a weaker suck and increased regurgitation as compared to her previous children. Physical examination is notable for underdevelopment, global spasticity, and hyperactive deep tendon reflexes. Microscopy reveals basophilic multinucleated macrophages with cytoplasmic inclusions.

| This child is suffering from what disorder? | Krabbe's disease (globoid leukodystrophy) |
| What is the deficient enzyme and mode of inheritance of this disorder? | Galactosylceramide $\beta$-galactosidase, autosomal recessive |
| What are the typical central nervous system (CNS) findings? | Demyelination of cerebral, cerebellar, and basal ganglier white matter |

A 4-year-old White male is brought to the pediatrician by his parents because of generalized "stiffness" and difficulty walking, especially climbing stairs, for the past several months. Physical examination reveals a child with a wide-based unsteady gait accompanied by ataxia. Deep tendon reflexes are exaggerated and Babinski's sign is elicited. Microscopy reveals brownish granules in oligodendrocytes upon staining with toluidine blue.

| This child is suffering from what disease process? | Metachromatic leukodystrophy (autosomal recessive) |
| What is this patient's enzyme deficiency? | Arylsulfatase A |
| In what additional organ will this patient show the aforementioned deposition? | Kidneys |

A recently adopted 2-year-old child of African decent is brought to the pediatric clinic by his Caucasian foster parents. They are concerned about his general appearance. The child appears generally cachectic with a large abdomen, depigmented skin and hair, and generalized pitting edema. The child is below the fifth percentile in height and weight.

| | |
|---|---|
| This child is suffering from what form of malnutrition? | Kwashiorkor (protein deprivation with normal total caloric intake) |
| What is the cause of the generalized pitting edema? | Hypoalbuminemia |
| What changes would be expected to be seen in the liver? | Fatty infiltration |

A 10-year-old White male is brought in by his parents for evaluation of his mental retardation. The boy has a long and narrow face, prominent ears, and enlarged testicles. The mother reports a possible history of mental retardation on her side of the family.

| | |
|---|---|
| This child is likely suffering from what disorder? | Fragile X syndrome |
| What is the etiology behind the mutation responsible for this condition? | Triple-nucleotide repeat in the FMR-1 gene on the X-chromosome |
| What condition is more commonly the cause of mental retardation in males? | Down Syndrome |

A 22-year-old male presents with complaints of recurrent sinus and upper respiratory tract infections. They have always been a problem but these infections have caused him to miss a substantial amount of work at his new job. On physical examination, it is noted that his heart is on the right side of his chest. Additionally, his liver is on the left side of his abdomen.

| | |
|---|---|
| This patient can be diagnosed with what condition? | Kartagener's syndrome |
| Why has this patient experienced recurrent sinus and upper respiratory tract infections? | The lack of dynein renders cilia of the sinuses and bronchi immotile, thus there is no mucus-clearing action |
| Why would this patient also be infertile? | His spermatozoa would be immotile as a result of the lack of dynein |

A 10-year-old White girl is brought in by her parents for evaluation of a skin disorder. The child has many freckles on her face, arms, and legs. In addition, she has telangiectasis along with areas of redness and hypopigmentation. The parents were told previously to limit her sun exposure as her skin is very sensitive to sunlight.

| | |
|---|---|
| What disorder does this child appear to be suffering from? | Xeroderma pigmentosum |
| What is the inheritance pattern and etiology of this disorder? | Autosomal recessive; impaired endonuclease excision repair mechanism of ultraviolet light-damaged DNA bases |
| Why were this child's parents told to limit their daughter's exposure to sunlight? | Sunlight sensitivity can predispose to epidermoid and basal cell carcinoma |

An 18-year-old Black male enlisted in the military service is vaccinated before being shipped off to central Africa. Several days later, he develops a fever and complains of weakness and fatigue. Physical examination reveals mild jaundice and slight nail bed pallor. On direct questioning, the man says that he was vaccinated against malaria amongst other illnesses.

| | |
|---|---|
| This patient is likely deficient in what enzyme? | Glucose-6-phosphate dehydrogenase |
| CBC and liver function tests (LFTs) would likely show what results? | Low hemoglobin, low hematocrit, reticulocytosis, elevated direct bilirubin |
| What is the inheritance pattern of this disease? | X-linked recessive |

A 1-year-old White girl is brought in by her parents because of lethargy, weakness, and yellowing of her skin. The child has palpable splenomegaly. CBC reveals microcytic anemia with dark red blood cells (RBCs) lacking any central pallor and increased numbers of reticulocytes. The father reports that he had been diagnosed with a blood disorder as a child.

| | |
|---|---|
| This child is suffering from what disease? | Hereditary spherocytosis |
| Why do the RBCs in this disease have an abnormal, spherical shape? | The RBC membranes lack spectrin, necessary to maintain the normal biconcave disk shape |
| What is the significance of the splenomegaly? | The abnormal shape of RBCs leads to higher rates of splenic sequestration and hemolysis with elevated direct bilirubin |

A 25-year-old girl complains of easy fatigability and weakness of approximately 3 years' duration. Physical examination reveals pallor, tachycardia, and cheilosis. She reports that her menses have been "heavy" as long as she can recall.

| | |
|---|---|
| This patient is likely suffering from what type of anemia? | Iron-deficiency anemia |
| What would microscopic examination with Prussian blue staining of her bone marrow likely show? | Erythroid hyperplasia with decreased bone marrow iron stores |
| What are possible treatments of this disorder? | Control menstrual blood loss, supplemental iron |

A newborn male is noted to be cyanotic a few hours after delivery. The child earlier had been circumcised using benzocaine ointment. On physical examination, the child is cyanotic with clear lungs bilaterally and normal heart sounds. Arterial blood gas (ABG) reveals normal oxygen partial pressure and a methemoglobin level of 20%.

| | |
|---|---|
| How does methemoglobin differ from normal hemoglobin? | Methemoglobin is an oxidized form and does not function as well as normal hemoglobin in carrying oxygen |
| Deficiency of what enzyme can also produce this disorder? | Nicotinamide adenosine dinucleotide (NADH) methemoglobin reductase |
| What is the treatment of choice for this disease? | Methylene blue, oxygen for acute symptoms |

A woman who survived a fire with traumatic full body burns is resting in the hospital in stable condition. Suddenly, the patient begins to use her accessory muscles of respiration and experiences dyspnea, tachypnea, rales, wheezing, and rhonchi bilaterally. CXR shows diffuse alveolar densities and air bronchograms.

| | |
|---|---|
| This patient is experiencing what syndrome? | Acute respiratory distress syndrome |
| What is the etiology behind this patient's syndrome? | Decreased surfactant production, neutrophil release of proteases, free radicals, and leukotrienes; lymphocyte and macrophage release of inter-leukin-1 and tumor necrosis factor |
| What is the immediate treatment of this disorder? | Mechanical ventilation, intensive care unit (ICU) care |

A 32-year-old nonsmoking female visits her doctor because of decreasing exercise tolerance. She says that she becomes short of breath after only a moderate amount of exercise. CBC shows increased hematocrit, pulmonary function test (PFT) shows a forced expiratory volume in the first second/forced vital capacity (FEV1/FVC) <80%, and electrocardiogram (ECG) shows right ventricular hypertrophy. CXR shows flattening of the diaphragm, decreased lung markings, and hyperlucent lung fields.

| | |
|---|---|
| This woman is suffering from what disorder? | $\alpha$-1-Antitrypsin deficiency |
| This disorder is associated with what type of emphysema? | Panacinar type (versus centrilobular type of cigarette smoking) |
| What other findings are expected on physical examination? | Barrel-shaped chest, decreased breath sounds bilaterally, hyperresonance to percussion, retardation of expiratory flow |

# Index

Page numbers followed by *f* indicate figures.